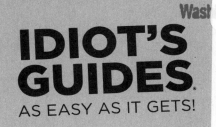

IDIOT'S GUIDES®

AS EASY AS IT GETS!

Gluten-Free Eating

by Elizabeth King Humphrey and Jeanette Hurt

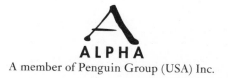

ALPHA

A member of Penguin Group (USA) Inc.

ALPHA BOOKS

Published by Penguin Group (USA) Inc.

Penguin Group (USA) Inc., 375 Hudson Street, New York, New York 10014, USA • Penguin Group (Canada), 90 Eglinton Avenue East, Suite 700, Toronto, Ontario M4P 2Y3, Canada (a division of Pearson Penguin Canada Inc.) • Penguin Books Ltd., 80 Strand, London WC2R 0RL, England • Penguin Ireland, 25 St. Stephen's Green, Dublin 2, Ireland (a division of Penguin Books Ltd.) • Penguin Group (Australia), 250 Camberwell Road, Camberwell, Victoria 3124, Australia (a division of Pearson Australia Group Pty. Ltd.) • Penguin Books India Pvt. Ltd., 11 Community Centre, Panchsheel Park, New Delhi—110 017, India • Penguin Group (NZ), 67 Apollo Drive, Rosedale, North Shore, Auckland 1311, New Zealand (a division of Pearson New Zealand Ltd.) • Penguin Books (South Africa) (Pty.) Ltd., 24 Sturdee Avenue, Rosebank, Johannesburg 2196, South Africa • Penguin Books Ltd., Registered Offices: 80 Strand, London WC2R 0RL, England

Copyright © 2014 by Penguin Group (USA) Inc.

International Standard Book Number: 978-1-61564-423-0
Library of Congress Catalog Card Number: 2013945264

16 15 14   8 7 6 5 4 3 2 1

Interpretation of the printing code: The rightmost number of the first series of numbers is the year of the book's printing; the rightmost number of the second series of numbers is the number of the book's printing. For example, a printing code of 14-1 shows that the first printing occurred in 2014.

Printed in the United States of America

Note: This publication contains the opinions and ideas of its authors. It is intended to provide helpful and informative material on the subject matter covered. It is sold with the understanding that the authors and publisher are not engaged in rendering professional services in the book. If the reader requires personal assistance or advice, a competent professional should be consulted.

The authors and publisher specifically disclaim any responsibility for any liability, loss, or risk, personal or otherwise, which is incurred as a consequence, directly or indirectly, of the use and application of any of the contents of this book.

Most Alpha books are available at special quantity discounts for bulk purchases for sales promotions, premiums, fund-raising, or educational use. Special books, or book excerpts, can also be created to fit specific needs. For details, write: Special Markets, Alpha Books, 375 Hudson Street, New York, NY 10014.

Publisher: *Mike Sanders*
Executive Managing Editor: *Billy Fields*
Executive Acquisitions Editor: *Lori Cates Hand*
Development Editorial Supervisor: *Christy Wagner*
Senior Production Editor: *Janette Lynn*

Cover Designer: *Laura Merriman*
Book Designer: *William Thomas*
Indexer: *Julie Bess*
Layout: *Ayanna Lacey*
Proofreader: *Laura Caddell*

This book is dedicated to my family and all those with whom I have shared a gluten-free meal and all those yet to come.
—Elizabeth

This book is dedicated to Ellen and Dick Haynes. —Jeanette

Contents

Appendixes

Introduction

If you're giving up gluten, you're not alone. More and more people are eliminating it from their diets. In fact, about 30 percent of American adults have expressed a desire to eat gluten free.

You might have a different reason for wanting to give up gluten than the next person, but most often, people say so long to gluten for medical reasons. Whether you suffer a gluten allergy, are gluten intolerant, or have been diagnosed with celiac disease, cutting out gluten is the only real option for getting better. That's what brought us to a gluten-free diet. Giving up gluten has not only cleared up some of our health issues, but it's also provided us with a healthier lifestyle. The same can be true for you, and in this book we show you how.

In the following chapters, we explain what exactly gluten is and some of the problems it can cause in your body. We also provide tips on choosing gluten-free grains while avoiding the ones that contain gluten and show you how delicious healthy, gluten-free, whole-food eating can be.

To make adopting a gluten-free diet even easier, we give you lots of advice on filling your pantry with fresh foods and gluten-free staples and offer guidance on preparing mouthwatering gluten-free meals and planning menus to help you stick with the program.

Dining out or eating at the homes of friends and family can present challenges to the gluten-free eater, so we give you suggestions on how to navigate life outside your home, including what to expect in restaurants and while traveling.

Eating gluten free doesn't mean you have to stop entertaining or throwing parties. In fact, this could be the perfect opportunity to create fabulous gluten-free menus to share with friends and family! And if you're a parent, we include a chapter on helping your child learn to navigate a gluten-free diet.

To assist you in finding new gluten-free dishes you can't wait to create and share, we include more than 90+ gluten-free recipes in the book. From breakfast to dessert, you'll never miss the gluten in these recipes.

Giving up gluten doesn't mean you give up fresh, delicious foods loaded with flavor. On the contrary, you'll discover new and tasty foods and dishes you'll wonder how you managed to get along without up to now!

Here's to healthy, gluten-free eating!

How This Book Is Organized

We've divided this book into four parts:

In **Part 1, Gluten and Your Body,** we explain what gluten is, where you find it, and why it causes problems for some people in the form of celiac disease, gluten intolerance, and gluten allergy. Because gluten seems to play a role in autoimmune disorders in addition to celiac disease, we also address that connection. We look at nutrition as well and explore how nutritionally sound your diet can be if you stop eating wheat and other gluten-containing grains. Finally, we take a look at the essential role whole foods can play in gluten-free eating.

Part 2, Gluten-Free First Steps, focuses on learning about what food you can eat on a gluten-free diet. We uncover where gluten often hides and discuss what safe grains, seeds, and beans you can substitute for gluten-based flours. Knowing what to look for and what to avoid helps you clean your kitchen of gluten and replenish your pantry with gluten-free goods. If you share your home with those who can eat gluten, we suggest ideas for gluten-free zones and additional kitchen equipment. We also share tips on navigating grocery and health food stores and tell you what to look for on food labels. Quick and easy meal options and gluten-free meal plans round out Part 2.

Part 3, Living a Gluten-Free Life, helps you safely eat gluten free outside your home at restaurants, fast-food joints, and while traveling. We also provide tips for entertaining gluten free and share advice on helping your kids thrive on a gluten-free diet, including tips for working with teachers and caregivers to keep your child safe.

In **Part 4, Gluten-Free Recipes,** we give you more than 90+ gluten-free recipes. From the first meal of the day to the last, we provide a variety of dishes to keep your stomach happy and gluten at bay.

At the back of the book, we've included further information you may find useful as you continue your gluten-free way of life. Please be sure to check out the glossary, additional resources, food log, and easy shopping list.

Extras

Throughout each chapter, we've included extra information, helpful tips, fun facts, and more. Here's what to look for:

> **DEFINITION**
>
> These sidebars provide explanations of terms you might not be familiar with.

FOOD FOR THOUGHT

Turn to these sidebars for fun facts and interesting bits of information.

GLUTEN GAFFE

These sidebars alert you to possible problems or pitfalls you may run across with gluten.

TASTY TIDBIT

These tips and timesavers help you survive and thrive on a gluten-free diet.

Throughout the book, we've also included special icons that indicate a recipe is vegan, kid friendly, or appropriate for those of you following a Paleo diet. Here's what to look for:

- 🥦 Vegan
- 😋 Kid friendly
- 🥑 Paleo diet friendly

Acknowledgments

We wish to give our heartfelt thanks to those who helped make this book possible: Marilyn Allen of Allen O'Shea Literary Agency; Executive Acquisitions Editor Lori Cates Hand and Development Editorial Supervisor Christy Wagner, for their guidance, encouragement, patience, and humor; Amie Valpone, editor in chief of TheHealthyApple.com; and the accommodating and super dietitian and educator Joan Clark-Warner, MS, RD, CDE. We would also like to thank our family and friends for their encouragement, understanding, and support while we were writing this book.

Elizabeth would like to give a special thanks to Ryanna Battiste, for her passion and community-building, and to Philip, for his unwavering support each day of this gluten-free journey.

Jeanette gives two thumbs way up to Damon Brown, her writing goal buddy, and Bec Loss, her website developer.

Special Thanks to the Technical Reviewer

Idiot's Guides: Gluten-Free Eating was reviewed by an expert who double-checked the accuracy of what you'll learn here, to help us ensure this book gives you everything you need to know about living a healthy, happy gluten-free life. Special thanks are extended to Trish Sebben-Krupka.

Trish is a chef specializing in vegan, vegetarian, sustainable, and health-supportive cooking. The author of *The Complete Idiot's Guide Greens Cookbook,* when she's not writing and editing, Trish enjoys teaching healthy cooking classes and cooking amazing family meals.

Trademarks

All terms mentioned in this book that are known to be or are suspected of being trademarks or service marks have been appropriately capitalized. Alpha Books and Penguin Group (USA) Inc. cannot attest to the accuracy of this information. Use of a term in this book should not be regarded as affecting the validity of any trademark or servicemark.

Gluten and Your Body

In Part 1, we get to know gluten and learn why it's a problem for some people. Then, we spend some time exploring gluten and its components to try to understand the disturbances they cause within your body. We look at gluten sensitivity, intolerance, and allergy and examine some of the disorders gluten can cause.

Then we shift gears and explain how gluten-free eating can help restore your health. We discuss the nutritional challenges you might face by not eating glutenous and fortified breads and clue you in to everything you *can* eat instead.

Understanding Gluten

Eliminating gluten is one of if not the only solution for better health if you're gluten intolerant, have been diagnosed with celiac disease, or have a wheat allergy.

One of the best ways to avoid gluten is to really understand what it is and where it's found. In this chapter, we explore gluten and help you understand that it's found in more foods than just wheat. We also look at what gluten can do to your body.

Even if you haven't been diagnosed as celiac or allergic to wheat, but you feel remarkably better when you avoid wheat-based products, the information in this chapter is worth your time to read.

In This Chapter

* Gluten—what is it?
* What gluten does to your body
* What other problems gluten causes
* Do your level of sensitivity to gluten

What Is Gluten, Exactly?

Gluten is a protein in wheat, rye, barley, and wheat derivatives. But this version of protein is a bit different from the protein you usually think of, the version found in meat or beans.

In cereal grains, protein is part of the structure of the food. This protein is gluten. Within wheat, gluten, which breaks down into gliadins and glutenins, is the main protein. Although the gliadins and glutenins are the two elements that form the gluten we refer to in this book, gliadin is the part of gluten that's toxic to gluten-sensitive people.

When you eat, your stomach and small intestine break down protein into single amino acids for your small intestine to digest. Gliadin is not easily digestible—even if you don't have celiac—and a part of it doesn't break down in your small intestine and the rest of your system. Your body then has a reaction to the gliadin and your small intestine villi start to be destroyed.

Celiac disease is thought to be caused by these toxic fragments of gliadin that don't break down. The peptide chain that creates gliadin is also what gives breads the elastic quality that we often miss in gluten-free breads. In rye, the gliadin-like protein is secalin. In barley, it's hordein.

You may have an allergy to gluten or an intolerance of it. Celiac disease is considered an intolerance. Which do you have? We look at the symptoms later in this chapter.

Is Gluten Only in Wheat?

Unfortunately, no. As mentioned, gluten is a protein that shows up in cereal grains, including wheat. So a type of this problematic gluten protein is also found in, for instance, barley and rye. However, you might not run into the same difficulties with those glutens as you do with wheat gluten because of their different structures.

Throughout the book, we use the term *gluten* to refer to the element in wheat, barley, rye, and wheat's relatives that consistently proves problematic for those suffering from gluten intolerance.

> **DEFINITION**
>
> **Gluten** is a protein found in wheat and other cereal grains.

Other similar foods might not present a problem for those with gluten issues, such as the gluten-containing spelt. (Not to confuse you, but spelt *might* be okay for someone who can't eat wheat. Consult with your health-care practitioner before diving into any spelt wraps though.) Generally, someone with a gluten intolerance is able to eat corn and rice.

Keeping track of which foods contain gluten and which are safe for you to eat can be terribly confusing. To make it simpler—and healthier—your medical practitioner might recommend you avoid wheat, barley, and rye.

He or she might have also told you to avoid oats because you can't be sure no cross-contamination occurred during the manufacturing process. This is a risk when a manufacturer processes foods that both do and don't contain gluten. But there is some good news: today, more and more brands are certifying they're gluten free so you can still eat your oats without fear of getting sick.

So What Exactly Is Wrong with Gluten?

After you chew and swallow a gluten-containing food, the gluten begins its trip through your digestive system, or your gastrointestinal tract. As food moves through your system, your body anticipates the delivery of some of the food's nutrients in your intestines. When the gluten arrives in your small intestines, if you have an allergy or an intolerance, your body starts setting off alarms.

Your body's immune system—half of which surrounds your digestive system—identifies the gluten as an attacker, and your white blood cells move in to conquer the invader. This battle creates inflammation in your intestines. When too much inflammation occurs, permeable areas open and start weakening your intestinal lining.

Normally, when food enters your small intestines, small particles of nutrients pass through the intestinal walls and into the blood stream. During the battle between your white blood cells and the gluten, however, the inflammation allows larger particles to pass through the lining of the small intestines.

If you continue to eat gluten, the proteins, bacteria, and other poisons leak from your intestines (also known as "leaky gut"), leading to even more inflammation. If you're predisposed, this cycle can leave your body susceptible to an autoimmune disorder, such as celiac disease, or other medical conditions.

With an allergy, histamines are present. Taking an antihistamine, such as Benadryl, can help quell an allergic reaction. With an intolerance, gliadin is recognized as an invader, but an antihistamine doesn't quiet the reaction. Undigested gliadin can remain in your intestine and cause even more inflammation.

Elizabeth's reaction to gluten is different from Jeanette's response to gluten, and our responses to gluten are different from what your response might be. Each person is different. Your genetic predisposition, your ability to handle stress, and the amount of "good" bacteria in your intestines all play a role in determining your reaction to gluten.

Irritable bowel syndrome, rashes, chronic fatigue, or ulcerative colitis may all be the result of one person's sensitivity to gluten. But for others, gluten intolerance may manifest as celiac disease, an autoimmune condition. Celiac disease is a gluten intolerance, but not all gluten intolerance is celiac disease.

Celiac disease is a genetic condition that destroys intestinal villi, the small nutrient absorbers in your small intestines. The villi help digest your food as well as provide a barrier against toxins entering your system. If your intestinal villi are okay, you probably suffer from gluten intolerance, not celiac disease.

At this time, the only way to know if your villi are okay is to have an endoscopic procedure that passes a small camera through your throat, stomach, and into your small intestine. A doctor takes pictures of your villi as well as takes a sample of your villi to see if any are flattened or otherwise damaged.

FOOD FOR THOUGHT

It's estimated that 1 in 10 Americans has a nonceliac form of gluten intolerance, which doesn't destroy the intestinal villi. The number of Americans with an autoimmune reaction to gluten, such as celiac disease, is 1 in 133.

An autoimmune disorder occurs when your body senses an intruder and antibodies go on the attack. This time it's not against a foreign agent but a part of your own body instead. In the case of those with celiac disease, what's attacked is the intestinal villi.

According to The University of Chicago Celiac Disease Center, celiac disease is "more frequent" if you have one of these autoimmune conditions:

- Type 1 diabetes mellitus
- Multiple sclerosis (MS)
- Hashimoto's thyroiditis
- Autoimmune hepatitis
- Addison disease
- Arthritis
- Sjögren's syndrome
- Idiopathic dilated cardiomyopathy
- IgA nephropathy

If you already have one of these medical conditions and haven't been diagnosed with celiac disease, you might want to contact your medical professional and request testing.

Symptoms to Watch For

Your body has probably been reacting to gluten in some manner, which is probably one of the reasons you're reading this book. Noting the way your body is responding to gluten is one of the ways your doctors can deduce what's been ailing you.

Your body responds to gluten with many symptoms, whether you have a nonceliac gluten sensitivity or celiac disease. The National Foundation for Celiac Awareness indicates there are almost 300 symptoms associated with celiac disease—with that many symptoms, celiac disease can often take years to diagnose. And because the symptoms aren't a histamine reaction, your symptoms might not show up immediately and can appear sometimes days after you consume a gluten-containing food.

According to the National Foundation for Celiac Awareness, if you have nonceliac gluten sensitivity or celiac disease, you may experience gastrointestinal symptoms and reactions in other parts of your body. You might experience the following:

- Abdominal pain

- Fatigue

- Headaches

- Tingling or numbness

- Brain fog

Keeping a food log (see Appendix D) is a good idea so you start tracking what you may be experiencing after eating certain foods. It will also help you target what you ate that brought on an adverse reaction. Trying a gluten-free challenge—where you eliminate foods with gluten for a period of 2 weeks or 30 days—could help, too.

Gluten Intolerance Symptoms

If you're gluten intolerant, you may experience these symptoms, which do not produce a quick histamine reaction:

- Diarrhea or constipation

- Fatigue

- Headaches

- Eczema or itchy skin

- Hypoglycemia

- Mental fog

- Autoimmune disorders, like Graves', lupus, Sjögren's syndrome, type 1 diabetes, or thyroiditis

- Joint or muscle pain

- … and almost 200 other issues, according to Dr. Stephen Wangen in *Healthier Without Wheat*

Gluten can be so insidious to your body that you could exhibit only a few, one, or even no symptoms before being diagnosed.

> **GLUTEN GAFFE**
>
> Children can exhibit other symptoms of gluten intolerance, including a failure to grow.

Food intolerance reactions, without triggering your body's histamines, may be delayed, but they are decidedly more complicated for your body. Intolerance can create inflammation, and, if you have the predisposition, could lead to your small intestine's villi flattening, which means they're not as capable of processing nutrients from your food. This can lead to malnutrition. When this condition is not treated—by avoiding gluten—then other diseases may develop. Sensitivity to gluten can lead to organ or tissue damage, as well as an overactive immune system.

Celiac Disease Symptoms

There are two types of gluten intolerance—celiac and nonceliac. For the majority of the book, we shorten the term to *gluten intolerance,* which we believe is applicable to the celiac and nonceliac forms. Celiac disease is a form of gluten intolerance.

You may hear *celiac disease* called *celiac sprue, tropical sprue,* or *gluten-sensitive enteropathy.* (Celiac sprue is how celiac disease was once referred to.) Some other diseases, such as tropical sprue and Crohn's disease, can also cause the small intestine villi to atrophy.

> **DEFINITION**
>
> **Celiac disease** is the genetic autoimmune disease that can be characterized by the destruction of villi in the small intestine as well as malnutrition. Its only treatment, to date, is the avoidance of gluten. Celiac disease has also been referred to as celiac sprue.

Celiac disease has a genetic component to it, but often some of the disease's symptoms lead to diagnoses of irritable bowel syndrome (IBS). In addition to the symptoms mentioned earlier as signs of intolerance, those with celiac disease can exhibit the following:

- Anemia
- Attention deficit disorder (ADD) or attention deficit hyperactivity disorder (ADHD)
- Fertility difficulties
- Migraines
- Dermatitis herpetiformis (a skin condition)
- Osteoporosis or osteopenia
- Depression
- Tooth enamel problems

To receive a diagnosis of celiac disease, you need to also exhibit the flattening of the villi. Genetic testing can also confirm the presence of genes that indicate the predisposition to celiac disease.

Gluten Allergy Symptoms

Celiac disease is not an allergy in the technical, medical sense. It's a genetic autoimmune disease. (If someone doesn't understand when you try to explain celiac disease, you may be tempted to explain that celiac disease is an allergy to gluten. Just be aware that celiac disease is not an allergy.)

An allergy to wheat or gluten will be triggered within a relatively short time—from within minutes to up to an hour. Basically, your body is trying to defend itself against a histamine reaction to the protein in the allergen.

If a person with an allergy to wheat consumes it, the physical response could be the following:

- Hives
- Throat itching or swelling
- Stomach cramping
- A drop in blood pressure
- Vomiting or diarrhea
- Asthma attack

Taking an antihistamine, such as Benadryl, should improve the wheat-allergic sufferer's near-immediate reaction.

As a lifelong peanut allergy sufferer, Elizabeth has experienced all of these symptoms when she's accidentally ingested peanuts. In fact, her anaphylaxis reaction can be so severe she may need to use emergency epinephrine or get hospitalization.

In comparison, Elizabeth's delayed reaction to eating gluten starts with lethargy, stomach cramps, and frequent bathroom visits. Her gluten reaction is not nearly as quick or immediately severe as her peanut reaction. Nonetheless, it's not very pleasant and has farther-reaching consequences.

What's in a Diagnosis?

The gold standard for diagnosing celiac is a biopsy of the small intestines. The small bowel biopsy or endoscopy indicates if you have damaged villi in your small intestine. However, if you plan to have a biopsy and have already stopped eating gluten, you'll need to return to eating gluten for a short period before undergoing the biopsy.

Without having a biopsy, genetic testing is available and can indicate if you have HLA-DQ2 and HLA-DQ8, the genes for celiac disease. You could have the genes, without full-blown celiac disease developed yet. But if you don't have the genes for celiac disease, the National Foundation for Celiac Awareness indicates that it's "nearly impossible" for you to develop celiac disease.

Because you need the genetic component to have the disease, some practitioners suggest testing for the HLA-DQ2 or HLA-DQ8 genes first, before having a biopsy. But if you've already given up gluten and aren't interested in returning to a glutenous diet, you should discuss genetic testing with your medical professional.

According to The University of Chicago Celiac Disease Center, there are no tests to confirm nonceliac gluten sensitivity.

However, the National Foundation for Celiac Awareness suggests your health-care professional could order an antibody screening for celiac. Some of the antibody tests for a suggested celiac blood panel are as follows:

- Anti-Tissue Transglutaminase (tTG-IgA)

- Total Serum IgA

- Anti-Endomysial Antibody (EMA-IgA)

You also may hear about gliadin—part of the glutenin and gliadin that makes up gluten—when discussing your gluten intolerance with your medical practitioner. Some may recommend the Anti-Gliadin (IgA and IgG) test, which looks at your gliadin antibodies to determine if they're elevated or not.

If you exhibit signs of a painful skin rash—dermatitis herpetiformis—your doctor may recommend a skin biopsy to confirm celiac disease.

A diagnosis can help determine the level of injury to your system. If you do have celiac disease, your medical practitioner can also watch for the development of other autoimmune diseases. Once you have one, you become susceptible to developing others.

 TASTY TIDBIT

> A diagnosis of celiac disease may provide, if you itemize, a medical expense tax deduction because the only treatment for celiac disease is to eat gluten-free foods. For example, if you buy gluten-free pasta for $5 and the glutenous version normally costs $1, you can deduct the $4 difference. Be sure to check with your tax professional to confirm how to deduct for celiac disease.

Treatments for Gluten Sensitivities

Clinical tests are underway for vaccines to treat celiac disease. Some of the drugs in development focus on gluten's penetration through the small intestine's walls and certain enzymes that will digest gluten, making it harmless to the stomach and small intestines.

At this time, however, the best and only advice for those with gluten sensitivities is to avoid gluten.

The Least You Need to Know

- Gluten is a protein found in wheat and other cereal grains.
- Gluten intolerances and allergies manifest in your body in different ways. Allergic reactions are generally more immediate than intolerance reactions.
- Gluten sensitivity may manifest as celiac disease, a genetic, autoimmune condition. Celiac disease is a gluten sensitivity, but not all gluten sensitivity is celiac disease.
- Currently, avoiding gluten is the only treatment for celiac disease, medicines are in development to treat gluten intolerances.

CHAPTER 2

Gluten-Free Nutrition

Eliminating gluten-containing foods and ingredients that have been making you sick is the only way to feel better if you have a gluten allergy or intolerance. But what, then, are you supposed to eat? Should you stop eating all grains and follow the Paleo diet? Or are there other alternatives, like eating fresh foods?

In this chapter, we discuss considerations you need to make in order to eat a healthful, balanced, gluten-free diet. It helps if you get in the right mind-set first. Instead of regarding this change as *restrictive,* look at it as a way to improve your overall lifestyle. Selecting foods that are naturally gluten free is a big first step. The rest will fall into place.

In This Chapter

- The importance of fresh, whole foods
- Understanding nutrition
- A look at vitamins and supplements
- What about Paleo?

Choosing Naturally Gluten-Free Foods

Clinical dietitian Joan Clark-Warner, MS, RD, CDE, notes: "Many problems that arise with a gluten-intolerance can be resolved with the right gluten-free diet approaches." That starts with your new food choices. When eating a gluten-free diet, opt for *whole foods* that are naturally gluten free whenever possible.

> **DEFINITION**
>
> A **whole food** is a food in its natural, unprocessed state. Fresh or frozen broccoli is a whole food, but broccoli with lemon pepper sauce or cheese sauce is not.

If you did nothing else, this would be a healthful way to approach eating and would keep you on a gluten-free path.

Eating Fresh Foods

Choose fresh first as often as you can. This means avoiding processed foods, and heading to the produce section first instead. Choose fresh whole foods, and buy the highest quality you can afford. Not only will the food be good for your body, it will taste better, too.

Start thinking of food in terms of the nutrition it can provide for your body. If you build your meals around good nutrition, you'll feel better, and your gut will begin healing from the damage gluten has caused. Remember, if you're gluten intolerant, your lower intestine is trying to heal itself, and the best way to facilitate this healing is through good, nutrient-rich foods.

Fruits and vegetables are naturally gluten free, and they're also naturally filled with antioxidants, vitamins, and minerals—all the good, nutritional building blocks that help heal your gut. If you can start focusing on them as the basis of your meals, your diet will naturally be healthier than it used to be, especially if you previously ate a lot of processed foods.

Eliminating Foods and Making Substitutions

You've been told to cut out gluten, but you really enjoy your lunch sandwich every day. Do you need to find something else to eat or just substitute the bread for gluten-free bread? The easiest solution is to find a good, gluten-free bread that you can substitute for your previously favorite carb. But you may also want to find other, gluten-free choices you can enjoy at lunchtime.

One thing we've both found is that gluten-free eating requires more planning. Not every restaurant has gluten-free options, and the quick, prepackaged foods we used to reach for when we wanted a quick snack or an easy dinner don't always fit in our new gluten-free diet.

You can easily substitute typical wheat products with starchy vegetables, such as potatoes, yucca, corn; or gluten-free grains, such as quinoa and rice. However, when making these substitutions, it's important to consider what you lose and what you gain.

GLUTEN GAFFE

Remember, just because a food doesn't contain gluten, that doesn't mean it's the healthiest choice for you and your body. A processed, lime-chipotle-flavored rice cracker is still a processed cracker, with little nutritional value.

Whole grains are good sources of the following:

- Protein

- Magnesium

- Manganese

- Zinc

- Copper

- Selenium

- B vitamins (B_1, B_2, B_3, B_9, and B_{12})

While starchy vegetables are good sources of these:

- Vitamin C

- Potassium

- Vitamin A

If you simply swap a whole grain for a starchy vegetable, you'll be missing out on some of the good things whole grains provide. Instead, try a mix of gluten-free whole-grain products and fresh, whole, starchy vegetables.

Many gluten-free products, especially breads, aren't as rich in fiber as whole-grain (wheat-based) products. To ensure you're getting enough fiber, you might want to increase your overall intake of fruits and vegetables. You also might want to look for more fiber-dense, gluten-free seeds and grains such as quinoa and buckwheat.

Also, consider the nutritional profile of the gluten-free vegetables you eat. A roasted sweet potato provides many more nutrients than french fries, a fried food that potentially contains additives. Although both are technically gluten free, the sweet potato is a whole food whereas the french fries are generally processed and often contain more than just the potato. Your roasted sweet potato—even a baked white potato—is more nutrient dense than french fries.

Be aware that as you change your eating habits, even though you're avoiding gluten, you need to continue to get a balance of vitamins and minerals from your foods.

 TASTY TIDBIT

Fresh fruits and vegetables, whole grains, nuts, and legumes—the world's healthiest populations rely on these staples. To learn more about populations that live long and healthy lives, check out *The Blue Zones: 9 Lessons for Living Longer from the People Who've Lived the Longest* by Dan Buettner.

Healthy Without Gluten

Eliminating gluten is the best step toward healing your body and feeling better. In the majority of cases, it's the *only* step suggested after a diagnosis of any kind of gluten sensitivity. But if you want to get healthier and stay healthier, it's important to not just avoid gluten, but to ensure your diet is nutritionally sound.

The Building Blocks of Nutrition

Carbohydrates, fat, and protein are the building blocks of nutrition. These elements are essential to human life. They provide the fuel your body needs, and you cannot survive without them.

Carbohydrates, which are interconnected sugar molecules, are a key source of energy. In your body, carbohydrates are synthesized into glucose. Carbohydrates and the glucose produced create energy for each cell.

Carbohydrates come in simple and complex varieties. The simple carbohydrates—fruit sugars—are easy for your body to break down. Complex carbohydrates—pasta, potatoes, grains, and rice—take longer to break down and give your body more fuel for a longer period. Complex carbohydrates, therefore, give your body more energy. In a balanced diet, the majority of your calories should come from good carbohydrates high in dietary fiber, not from candies and cookies, which also have carbs.

Fats are, like carbs, part of your body's fuel. Unlike carbohydrates, though, fats don't dissolve in water, so they can slow your digestion. Fat, in terms of its weight, provides twice the energy of carbohydrates. And fats usually taste good (think butter), which is why we add them to many foods. Your body can store fat in your body's fat cells indefinitely, but it's unable to store carbs for as long. Carbs store in your body for a day or two, so your body looks to carbs first, before fat and fatty acids.

Avocados, salmon, sardines, nuts, seeds, and olive oil provide healthy fat for your body.

Twenty percent of the daily caloric intake of the standard American diet (SAD) comes from *protein*. Although protein is important, it comes after carbs and fats in order of importance.

> **DEFINITION**
>
> **Protein** refers to the collection of 20 amino acids your body needs to survive. A *complete* protein includes all 20 amino acids; an *incomplete* protein is missing one or more of the amino acids. *Complementary* proteins refer to foods that are incomplete proteins separately but provide an excellent protein when combined.

Your body takes the protein in beans, nuts, fish and other meats, eggs, and dairy and breaks it into smaller molecules, called amino acids. Your body reaches for the protein in your body if you don't have fat or carbs to provide energy. It is the last of the three building blocks your body needs for your optimal health.

Get Some Color in Your Diet

For optimal health, your meals should consist of colorful foods. When Elizabeth first consulted with a health-care provider about her gluten intolerance, she was given a brightly colored food wheel. The wheel provided a visual example of the foods we should regularly include in our diets, broken down by color of food. Eggplants and plums, for example, are situated in the purple section of the wheel.

By eating a rainbow of differently colored foods every day, you tend to eat more whole foods and, therefore, reap more of the foods' nutrients.

> **FOOD FOR THOUGHT**
>
> It's not always easy to eat a variety of colorful fruits and vegetables every day. To help with this, the U.S. Centers for Disease Control and Prevention maintains a website (fruitsandveggiesmatter.gov) where you can plug in your weight and amount of physical activity you get and receive a recommendation of what fruit and vegetables you should eat daily. As long as you're changing your diet to eliminate gluten, why not try to boost your colorful fruit and vegetable intake?

Here are some fruits and vegetables to get you started thinking about ways to incorporate more color into your diet:

- Red: Red apples, red peppers, beets, radishes, raspberries, pink grapefruit, red grapes, watermelon

- Orange or yellow: Yellow apples, peaches, butternut squash, yellow peppers, persimmons, pumpkin, tangerines

- Green: Green apples, honeydew melon, artichokes, avocados, green peppers, limes, green beans, green onions, kale

- Blue or purple: Blackberries, blueberries, raisins, eggplant, figs, plums

- White: Bananas, cauliflower, potatoes, jicama, mushrooms, onions, ginger, garlic

And that's just a quick sampling. We're sure you can come up with other colorful whole foods to fill your plate.

Essential Vitamins

Understanding vitamins—how they function and in what foods they're found—is particularly important for you if you're gluten intolerant. Vitamins are an essential part of your ability to process food and they also boost your body's abilities. The beta-carotene in carrots, for example, transforms into vitamin A to promote eye health.

Because of the way gluten blocks the absorption of important vitamins and minerals, those with gluten intolerance might be deficient in many of the B vitamins, especially vitamin B_{12}, vitamin K, vitamin D, protein, calcium, and trace nutrients. Gluten-intolerant folks might also benefit from anti-inflammatory nutrients such as omega-3 fatty acids and vitamin C, which can help with gastrointestinal inflammation.

Providing your body with adequate vitamins is one of the most important reasons for increasing the amount of whole foods you eat. Whole foods are full of vitamins and minerals, and your body can absorb them more easily than those you take in a pill form.

Believe it or not, cooking can sometimes reduce the amount of vitamins in foods. To retain the vitamins in the foods you prepare, follow these guidelines:

- Don't overcook vegetables or fruits.

- Blanch or steam foods.

- When boiling, don't overboil, and do not overcrowd.

TASTY TIDBIT

Don't throw out the water left over after boiling vegetables! You can add it to smoothies and soups to add a nutritional punch.

More Gut Healers

Forty nutrients, including vitamins, are critical to your body. Two of these are commonly recommended to help the digestive tract, especially the small intestine, heal itself:

- L-glutamine

- Omega-3

L-glutamine—found in meat, dairy products, beans, cabbage, and spinach—is one of the 20 amino acids. Among other things, it provides fuel for your small intestine and strengthens your immune system. This is why it's especially beneficial to those with celiac disease.

Omega-3 fatty acids help reduce inflammation in the small intestine. Fish oil supplements contain omega-3s. Flaxseeds are also high in omega-3, and ground flaxseeds are a great way to add fiber and nutrition. Just sprinkle the powdered seeds in your smoothies, add them to your baked goods, or top them on your cereal. Other sources of omega-3s include fish (not just fish oils); hemp seeds; dark, leafy vegetables; and walnuts.

FOOD FOR THOUGHT

The best vitamin supplements are those derived from actual, whole foods, so read labels. Some supplements are less effectively absorbed than others, so it's a good idea to first consult with your health-care provider to determine which vitamin supplements are right for you.

Nutritional Malabsorption

Before you gave up gluten, your gluten-intolerant body—specifically your digestive tract—might have been reacting to food by not absorbing its nutrients. This is called *nutritional malabsorption.*

If your body isn't absorbing nutrients properly, you may experience symptoms such as the following:

- Inability to grow or gain weight
- Anemia, including deficient in vitamin B_{12} or iron
- High cholesterol
- Vitamin D deficiency
- Tooth enamel problems
- Hypoglycemia, or low blood sugar
- Depression
- Migraines
- Loss of bone density
- Exhaustion and reduction of strength

The good news is, you can alleviate the nutritional malabsorption caused by gluten intolerance. Here are some suggestions:

- Eat whole foods, and forego processed foods.
- Supplement with a multivitamin that includes minerals.
- Eat smaller meals and snacks throughout your day, and don't miss any meals, to improve the nutrients your body absorbs.
- Take time to chew your food thoroughly.

If you've eliminated gluten and you experience bloating, take notice of what you ate and investigate possible reasons for your reaction. Keeping a food diary—writing down what you eat and what your reactions are to certain foods—can help you discover what's causing you problems. In some cases, it can help you discover hidden sources of gluten that have been contaminating your food.

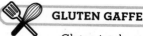 **GLUTEN GAFFE**

Gluten intolerance isn't just a stomach or intestinal problem; it can lead to almost 200 difficulties and physical ramifications.

The Paleo Diet

Often when there's a discussion of gluten-free eating, there's also a mention of the Paleo diet. Paleo, short for *Paleolithic,* recommends a diet similar to those our hunter-gatherer ancestors ate, before cultivation introduced large quantities of grains, legumes, and sugars to our diets. Paleo books abound with the benefits of the diet, including weight loss, reduced inflammation, and decreased risk of diseases that seem rampant in today's society.

Those who follow the Paleo diet avoid sugar, vegetable oils, and gluten—that's right: no wheat, rye, barley, oats, or other grains. In this way, it's obviously similar to gluten-free eating.

However, the Paleo diet also recommends you avoid legumes, which include peanuts, beans, and soy. Corn is also on the list of items to dodge. These are acceptable and encouraged ingredients in a gluten-free diet. As someone with a gluten intolerance, you *could* eat a Paleo diet, but you'd be limiting yourself to avoiding more than just foods with gluten.

The Paleo diet does provide great suggestions for meal ideas. It encourages eating the following:

- Fruits

- Vegetables

- Meats

- Fish

- Eggs

- Healthy fats such as avocados and palm, coconut, or olive oils

While it recommends avoiding the following:

- Sugars—only the rare use of honey or maple syrup is acceptable

- Processed and vegetable oils, such as canola, corn, and soybean

- Legumes, which includes peanuts

- Dairy, although some who follow the Paleo diet may eat dairy from high-quality, grass-fed sources

Although it's not a no- or low-carbohydrate diet, you could certainly restrict your carbohydrate intake as well.

While the Paleo diet is a good place to turn for gluten-free recipes, keep in mind that it may not necessarily be the best diet for you. Many health professionals believe a diet that includes a variety of whole foods, including dairy and legumes, is best.

Even if you don't plan to adopt the Paleo lifestyle, you can probably breathe easily if you're invited to friends' homes if they follow the Paleo diet. (But always make dinner hosts aware of your gluten intolerance, just in case.)

The Least You Need to Know

- Gluten-free does not automatically mean "healthful."
- Focus on eating a wide variety of whole foods, including fruits and vegetables of all colors, to get the nutrients you need.
- Gluten-intolerant people are often deficient in certain vitamins. Consult with your health-care provider to determine what supplements you may need to take.
- The Paleo diet is gluten free, but it also avoids vegetable oils, sugars, dairy, and legumes—all of which can be part of a gluten-free diet.

Gluten-Free First Steps

In Part 2, we show you how rich your diet can be without gluten. We explore all the grains, seeds, flours, and thickeners you can eat as you eliminate gluten and show you how to make successful substitutions for wheat flour.

Equally important as what you can eat, we highlight what you shouldn't eat. We also show you how to spot hidden gluten in foods and drinks as you shop.

Part of gluten-free *eating* means gluten-free *cooking,* so we help you prepare your kitchen. We offer recommendations on what to get rid of, what to keep, and how to manage your gluten-free lifestyle in a house where gluten may still lurk.

The idea of shopping for gluten-free foods might seem overwhelming to you right now, but we've got that covered, too. We share lots of tips and tricks for navigating the grocery store and even help you plan a 2-week menu plan for dozens of delicious gluten-free meals—using many of the recipes in Part 4!

CHAPTER 3

What to Eat

When you first learned about restricting your gluten intake, you probably thought more about what you *couldn't* eat than what you *can*. This is a natural reaction because you've likely been eating wheat, barley, rye, and oats without question for years.

Eating gluten-free isn't just about limitations. That's why we want to introduce you to some of the many ingredients you *can* eat as you start your gluten-free journey. You may be avoiding gluten, but you're not avoiding great-tasting food.

In this chapter, we review a handful of gluten-free grains and seeds, flours, and thickeners, most of which are readily available at your local grocery. You learn how to use these ingredients singly and in combination to replace the gluten-based ingredients you're used to.

Avoiding gluten may not be the only limitation in your diet, so we've included suggested substitutions for eggs and lactose as well. Some of these items may be completely new to you, whereas you might be familiar with others. In any case, let's jump in and start exploring.

In This Chapter

- Gluten-free seeds and grains
- Exploring gluten-free flours
- Alternatives to wheat-based thickeners
- Making gluten-free substitutions

Sensational Seeds and Gluten-Free Grains

Botanically speaking, seeds and grains are different. Technically, a grain is a fruit with a single seed fused, and a seed is an egg or ovule of a plant with a plant embryo inside. Many times—even on food labels—the terms *seed* and *grain* are used interchangeably.

Whether you call them *seeds* or *grains,* you should get to know the great gluten-free foods in the following sections.

Amaranth

Amaranth is a well-balanced protein powerhouse. According to the Whole Grains Council (wholegrainscouncil.org), amaranth isn't a true grain, but it's often referred to as a grain thanks to its uses and nutritional profile. This small, yellowish seed is loaded with lots of amino acids and does particularly well in the *lysine* department. It's easy to cook and can be used in a wide variety of foods.

> **DEFINITION**
>
> **Lysine** is one of the 20 essential amino acids that provide the building blocks for human protein. Of those, several are required for adults—isoleucine, leucine, lysine, methionine, phenylalanine, threonine, tryptophan, and valine; histidine can be among the essentials, too. Normally grains do not have much lysine, but in this case, amaranth and buckwheat do.

Amaranth has been cultivated since the time of the Aztecs, but it was relatively unknown in the United States until the 1970s, when it gained popularity for its versatility and health benefits.

Amaranth grain and flour are available in many health food stores. Amaranth flour is often used in quick breads, cookies, and muffins, and amaranth seeds may be used in granola-type snack bars. Puffed amaranth can be used for breakfast cereal or for a side dish. You can find many amaranth recipes, including soups, stews, and drinks, on the Amaranth Institute's website (amaranthinstitute.org).

When shopping for amaranth flour, try Arrowhead Mills Organic Whole Grain, Bob's Red Mill Organic, and Nuts.com. You can find amaranth seed from these sources, too.

Buckwheat

Buckwheat, which has a slightly nutty taste, is probably the most misunderstood of the wheat replacements. A relative of rhubarb, buckwheat has "wheat" in its name, but it's actually not a wheat. It's a fruit seed. Buckwheat is naturally gluten free, is one of the best-known sources of complex carbohydrates, and has high levels of all eight amino acids required for adults.

You may run across recipes that use buckwheat flour, such as pancakes and waffles. Unroasted buckwheat *groats* and kasha, which is roasted buckwheat groats, are often cooked like rice and can be eaten for breakfast or added to soups and stuffing.

> **DEFINITION**
>
> **Groats** is the term used for hulled cereal grains, such as oats, wheat, barley, and rye, as well as hulled grainlike seeds such as buckwheat. Groats are whole grains and are often used in soups and porridges.

Now that you know it's gluten free, you'll find all sorts of uses for buckwheat. Even the hulls can be used for filling pillows.

A few brands of buckwheat flour to look for include Arrowhead Mills Organic Whole Grain, Bob's Red Mill Organic, and Nuts.com.

Corn

Nearly a quarter of the world derives nutrition from corn, according to the Whole Grains Council. High in vitamin A, corn is used in a wide variety of food products. You may be accustomed to eating sweet corn during its summer peak, but corn appears in many other forms as well:

- Grits
- Polenta (made from cornmeal)
- Hominy
- Cornstarch

Soaking corn kernels in an alkaline solution, often lime water, increases corn's calcium and provides for more bioavailable B vitamins. The kernels are then dried and ground into flour, resulting in *masa harina*. You can find this flour, which is often used in making tortillas, in grocery stores.

Cornmeal, which is ground dried corn kernels, and corn flour, which is finely ground cornmeal, are used in many gluten-free products. You can use cornmeal and corn flour for quick breads, yeast breads, muffins, and piecrusts.

Bob's Red Mill Organic and Nuts.com are two good sources of corn flour and cornmeal.

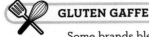

GLUTEN GAFFE

Some brands blend cornmeal with glutenous flours, so always check the label when you're buying cornmeal and corn flours. Cornbread mixes, in particular, often contain more than just corn and introduce contaminants.

Millet

Millet, like many of the other grains and seeds we're reviewing, has been around for thousands of years. In fact, millet may have been used to make polenta before the Italians started using corn for that dish.

Of the several varieties of millet—pearl, foxtail, proso, and finger—pearl is what you'll find most often in American grocery stores. Even though millet holds the sixth place in the list of important grains globally, you may have only seen this small, round seed in birdseed in the United States.

Millet is high in antioxidants and magnesium and is considered a great food for reducing inflammation. Including it in a breakfast porridge is a great way to work it into your diet. Always rinse millet before using it.

Look for Arrowhead Mills Organic Whole Grain, Bob's Red Mill Organic, and Nuts.com millet flour and seed. Arrowhead Mills also makes a puffed millet.

Quinoa

Another ancient "grain," quinoa (*KEEN-wah*) is related to beets, spinach, and chard. Small and round, the tiny quinoa seed resembles millet. Quinoa is a complete protein and packs an incredible nutritional punch. It's often recommended for decreasing the risk of diabetes.

FOOD FOR THOUGHT

The Incas considered quinoa sacred and the "mother of all grains." Because of the rituals surrounding quinoa, Spanish explorers destroyed the quinoa fields. However, wild quinoa continued to grow. In the 1970s, quinoa started its resurgence.

The popularity of quinoa has grown in recent years, and different varieties have started appearing on the U.S. market, including red, yellow, and black quinoa. Quinoa flakes, flour, and pasta are also becoming more readily available.

Many stores sell whole quinoa seeds in the bulk foods section, which is a great option for budget-minded shoppers or if you want to try just a small amount. However, those who suffer from Celiac disease should avoid purchasing quinoa (and other bulk items) due to the risk of cross-contamination from other bulk bins.

A few brands of quinoa seeds and flour are Ancient Harvest, Bob's Red Mill Organic, and Nuts. com.

Rice

Rice is a gluten-free food used in dozens of cuisines throughout the world. There are thousands of varieties of rice to choose from, but you're probably most familiar with white rice—it's brown rice without its bran. Rice classifications include the size of the grain (long, medium, and short), as well as the color (brown, white, black, and red). Each color provides different antioxidants.

Unlike some of the other seeds and grains we've covered, rice does not provide a significant amount of protein. However, it is a good source of calcium, iron, niacin, and riboflavin. Brown rice ranks higher than wheat in terms of carbohydrate content and consists of more than two-thirds starch.

You might think of rice as just a side dish for dinners, but it's easy to incorporate into other meals, too. Rice porridge is a popular breakfast food in many countries, and rice flours—white, brown, and sweet—are frequently used in gluten-free baking. (Sweet rice is not rice with added sweetener, but a short-grained, sticky rice.)

Many brands of white rice flour are available, including Arrowhead Mills Organic Whole Grain, Bob's Red Mill Organic, Ener-G, Now, and Nuts.com. When shopping for brown rice flour, try Arrowhead Mills Organic Whole Grain, Bob's Red Mill Organic, Lundberg Family Farms, and Nuts.com. Sweet rice flour, also called Mochiko, is available from Bob's Red Mill, Ener-G, Koda, and Nuts.com.

 GLUTEN GAFFE

Rice is a great gluten-free food, but be careful not to consume more than three servings a week. A study published in November 2012 showed that rice and rice products contain low levels of arsenic, which could increase other health risks. The report recommended rinsing raw rice before cooking, using 6 cups water to 1 cup rice, and draining the water after the rice is cooked.

Sorghum

Sorghum, another grain that's thousands of years old, is a true cereal grain. Sorghum has gained popularity with those avoiding gluten because it's high in antioxidants and low on the glycemic scale.

Like many of the grains and seeds we've covered, sorghum can be used in flour form or whole seed form. The flour can be a substitute for wheat flour—start with recipes that don't rely entirely on wheat, and experiment. Because sorghum doesn't contain gluten, it needs a binding agent, such as xanthan gum. Some say sorghum has a sweeter taste than other flours; some say it has a neutral taste. Try it and decide for yourself.

Bob's Red Mill Organic and Nuts.com offer sorghum flour.

FOOD FOR THOUGHT

Sorghum is the third top grain crop in the United States, but the majority of sorghum is used to feed livestock.

Teff

Although it doesn't sound very appetizing, teff is a hearty grass that manages to grow in some not-so-hospitable climates. Teff (also spelled *tef*) is a small grain and difficult to process. The tiny, darkish-red grain packs in the calcium—1 cup grain contains 123 milligrams—and vitamin C.

Teff is available in whole grain form or as a flour. As a flour, it sometimes appears in blends of flours for baking purposes. Teff flour works well with bread recipes and cookies. You can prepare the grain form as a side dish or use it as a thickening agent.

Guar gum and xanthan gum provide binding for gluten-free baking. Add $^1/_2$ teaspoon xanthan gum or guar gum per 1 cup blended flours for cookies, muffins, and cakes. For yeast breads, add 1 teaspoon per cup.

Two brands of teff flour and grain are Bob's Red Mill Organic and Nuts.com.

Fantastic Flours

In this section, we take a look at some of the delicious flours you can use in gluten-free cooking and baking. As you start exploring cookbooks, you'll notice that some are devoted to single flours, such as almond. We've tried a lot of these flours—Elizabeth really enjoys baking with almond flour and coconut flour. She also likes using chickpea flour.

FOOD FOR THOUGHT

Gluten-free flours made from dried and milled grape seeds and grape skins have entered the market. You could have a little Cabernet flour in with your sandwich bread or a Chardonnay flour with your piecrusts. Cabernet, Merlot, Chardonnay, Sauvignon, and Riesling provide omega fatty acids, potassium, and vitamin A.

Almond Flour

Almond flour is milled from almonds without their skins. Almonds provide antioxidants along with potassium, magnesium, niacin, alpha-tocopherol, calcium, and iron. Almonds also help steady your blood sugar, are high in protein, and contain good fats that could help with cholesterol.

Almond flour is great to use in bread and cookie recipes.

When shopping for almond flour, try Bob's Red Mill Organic, Honeyville, Trader Joe's, and Nuts. com. Some brands distinguish their almond flour as fine and very fine. You may notice that some recipes call for one or the other.

Chickpea Flour

Move over, grains, and make room for legumes. Chickpea flour, or garbanzo bean flour, has higher protein content than that of grain flour and is good as a thickener. It also appears as *gram, besan,* and *chana dal.*

Chickpea flour is great to use in breads, but it can also be used to make falafel patties and to coat foods before you fry them.

A few brands of chickpea flour to look for are Authentic Foods, Bob's Red Mill Organic, and Nuts.com.

Coconut Flour

Coconut flour is gaining in popularity. Even if you don't like coconut, consider the flour because it doesn't have a coconut flavor when used. Made from dried and defatted coconut, the flour is less expensive than almond flour. However, it is important to note that this flour requires using a lot more liquid than other flours. Some chefs recommend using double the amount of liquid in a recipe if you use coconut flour.

Coconut flour is good for pancakes and waffles, but it also can be especially good in some cake recipes.

A few brands of coconut flour to try are Bob's Red Mill Organic, Coconut Secret, Let's Do … Organic, Nutiva, and Nuts.com.

Fava Bean Flour

Fava beans are used to create this earthy-tasting flour. Fava beans, which look similar to lima beans, are also called horse beans, faba beans, or broad beans.

Some people love using this flour in breads and pizzas.

A few brands of fava bean flour are Barry Farms, Bob's Red Mill Organic, and Nuts.com.

 FOOD FOR THOUGHT

Beans used for flours are dried and treated to help minimize any bloating. The beans are then milled into flour.

Garfava Flour

Garbanzo bean flour, another name for chickpea flour, is blended with fava bean flour to create this rather nutty-tasting flour that stands up well when combined with other gluten-free flours.

Because of its high protein content, garfava flour can be great for bread baking, but many chefs recommend combining it with a lighter flour like sorghum or millet.

Garfava, which also sells by the name of garbanzo fava flour, is manufactured by Authentic Foods, Bob's Red Mill Organic, and Nuts.com.

Hazelnut Flour

Baking something with chocolate? Consider using hazelnut flour, which helps deepen the taste of the chocolate. Pastries, cakes, and cookies often contain hazelnuts, and some gluten-free products are made with hazelnuts.

When cooking, use hazelnut flour to enrich the taste and texture of baked goods, especially cakes and cookies.

Bob's Red Mill and Nuts.com offer hazelnut flour, which is one of the more expensive nut flours.

GLUTEN GAFFE

Replacing glutenous flours with nut flours can present other problems. Many gluten-intolerant people report problems with other dietary allergens—nuts included. Be careful when sharing your nut-flour goodies, and be sure the recipients are aware they contain nut flours. The good news is that most nut flours can be seamlessly swapped with other nut flours in recipes.

Pecan Flour

Maple and pecan seem like a match, especially when baking gluten free. You can pair these flavors by using pecan flour, or pecan meal, along with maple syrup in baked goods. Pecan flour looks like ground flaxseeds.

Pecan flour is nice in piecrusts and breads. Some use it as a coating for meats.

Shop for Angelina's Gourmet, Barry Farm, and Nuts.com brands of pecan flour.

Potato Flour

Potato flour (sometimes labeled "potato starch flour") is made from the entire cooked potato and really absorbs water, which helps it act as a binder when you use it in baked goods. You should only use potato flour in small amounts; too much potato flour in a recipe, and it can become gummy and heavy.

Potato flour is generally not a good standalone flour because it has a distinctive potato flavor. Although some bakers like the moist texture of baked goods made with potato flour, others combine potato flour with other gluten-free flours.

A few brands of potato flour are Authentic Foods, Barry Farm, Bob's Red Mill Organic, Ener-G, and Nuts.com.

TASTY TIDBIT

Potato flour and potato starch are not interchangeable. Potato flour is made from the entire cooked potato, while potato starch is made from dehydrating the peeled potato. Unlike potato flour, potato starch won't absorb a lot of water unless you heat it, as in a sauce or gravy.

When buying potato bread products, be sure to check the labels. "Potato bread" often contains wheat and wheat by-products.

Soy Flour

Soy flour, often used in baked goods and to help thicken gravies, is made from milling roasted soybeans. The flour is rich in *isoflavones,* but if you're using this flour to replace your whole-wheat flour, substitute up to $^1/_4$ in your flour blend. Also be aware that soy is considered one of the eight main allergens, and those with gluten intolerance may be sensitive to soy as well.

Use soy flour as a thickener, to add protein to savory entrées, and in baked goods. Soy flour is often used in combination with gluten-free flours.

Arrowhead Mills and Nuts.com offer soy flour.

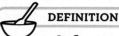

> **DEFINITION**
>
> **Isoflavones,** also called phytoestrogens, are plant estrogens found in soybeans, according to the Soyfoods Council. Isoflavones are associated with reducing inflammation.

Whole-Bean Flour

Romano beans are used to create whole-bean flour, which has a robust taste. If you can't find whole-bean flour, another bean flour, such as soybean flour, would be a decent substitute.

Romano bean flour can be used in bread baking.

El Peto is the only brand we found that sells whole-bean or romano bean flour. Another product you may see is Barry Farm's white bean flour, which may be an adequate substitute, but it's not one we've tried.

Terrific Thickeners

Wheat flour is often used as a *thickening agent.* Now that you're eating gluten free, you'll need a substitute to help thicken sauces and gravies and help bind ingredients when baking. The following thickeners can fill the bill nicely.

> **DEFINITION**
>
> **Thickening agents** are starches that change the viscosity of liquids. A gluten-free thickening agent—such as arrowroot, cornstarch, or tapioca starch—helps bind together liquids or make baked goods taste lighter.

Check your recipe, but often a starch reacts better when it's mixed with cold water before hitting the hot liquid.

Arrowroot

Arrowroot is made from a tropical tuber and has two times the thickening power of wheat flour. This fine white powder is tasteless and clear and thickens at a lower temperature than cornstarch and wheat.

Arrowroot is especially great when needing to thicken a fruit sauce or filling.

Look for arrowroot sold by such brands as Authentic Foods, Barry Farm, Bob's Red Mill Organic, Spicely, and Nuts.com. McCormick also makes arrowroot, which you can find in small jars in the spice section of the grocery store.

Cornstarch

Cornstarch, like arrowroot, is a very fine, white starch. It's often mixed with other flours in recipes for breads. Cornstarch is not the go-to thickener when a recipe also contains lemon juice, however; because the acidity of a citrus fruit will interfere with its thickening capabilities. Tapioca starch would be better.

Cornstarch is more readily available than some other thickeners. A few brands to look for are Bob's Red Mill Organic, Frontier, Let's Do … Organic, Nuts.com, and Rapunzel.

Potato Starch

Potato starch is made from the starch of the potato. It has a fine, powdery texture and helps make gluten-free baked goods moister.

Shop for brands such as Barry Farm, Bob's Red Mill Organic, Ener-G, Frontier, Manischewitz, and Nuts.com.

Tapioca Starch or Tapioca Flour

Tapioca starch (also called tapioca flour or cassava flour) is a great thickener for foods with a high acid content, such as fruit pie fillings.

A few brands of tapioca starch or tapioca flour to look for include Authentic Foods, Barry Farm, Bob's Red Mill Organic, Ener-G, Let's Do … Organic, Now, and Nuts.com.

Guar Gum

Guar gum is frequently used as an additive in manufactured gluten-free foods. It also serves as a thickening agent and a replacement for gluten. Guar gum is made from a plant in the legume family.

Guar gum can be found from Authentic Foods, Barry Farm, Bob's Red Mill Organic, Now, and Nuts.com.

> **GLUTEN GAFFE**
>
> Guar gum can act as a laxative in some people. When you start using it, do so in moderation to determine if it's right for you. Xanthan gum is slippery when wet, so work with it on a dry counter.

Xanthan Gum

Xanthan (*ZAN-than*) gum is made from fermented corn sugar, or glucose. Xanthan gum helps give baked goods volume and is often used as an additive in manufactured gluten-free foods because it performs similarly to gluten.

A few brands of xanthan gum to try include Authentic Foods, Barry Farm, Bob's Red Mill Organic, Ener-G, Hodgson Mills, Now, and Nuts.com.

Many gluten-free baking recipes call for xanthan gum or guar gum because they help the cakes and cookies keep from crumbling.

Smart Substitutions

Now that you know a little more about the many gluten-free flours available, you might be wondering how you can incorporate these new ingredients into your favorite recipes. In this section, we share some tips for making gluten-free substitutions.

Often those who have issues with gluten also exhibit problems with eggs and lactose, so we've included some ideas for replacing them, too.

Re-creating familiar flavors will take some experimentation, but you may end up discovering new tastes to enjoy.

Wheat Flour Substitutions

To create your own wheat flour substitution, *Living Without* magazine suggests creating an all-purpose flour by combining the following:

- $1/2$ cup rice flour (brown or white) or sorghum flour
- $1/4$ cup of a starch, such as tapioca
- $1/4$ cup cornstarch or potato starch

Alternatively, 1 cup corn flour, potato flour, or tapioca flour can be used in place of the same amount of wheat flour. But because none of these contain gluten, you'll want to blend the various flours along with a thickening agent like xanthan gum or guar gum.

Also keep in mind that gluten-free baked goods need about a third more baking soda or baking powder.

Once you start experimenting with different flours, you'll get a better idea of how you can combine them. Of course, prepackaged all-purpose gluten-free flour has worked out all the kinks, so you could easily use the preblended kind for substitutions. Follow the package directions, and note that the manufacturer may have already added guar gum or xanthan gum as a binding agent. Even if one of the gums has already been added to the flour you're using in a recipe, it's a good idea to add xanthan gum or guar gum if the recipe calls for it.

> **FOOD FOR THOUGHT**
>
> Mesquite flour, made from the dried beans of the mesquite tree, is another gluten-free flour you might want to check out. It acts as a flour or as a spice, with its sweet and earthy, almost nutty flavor.

Eggless Considerations

If you're also allergic to eggs, a few substitutions are available. Applesauce is one of the easier replacements to use. For each egg you want to replace in a recipe, use $1/4$ cup applesauce. You also can use 2 tablespoons arrowroot or potato starch without water to replace 1 egg. Another great replacement is ground flaxseeds; 2 tablespoons ground flaxseed mixed with 3 tablespoons water equals 1 egg in recipes.

Ener-G Egg Replacer, a vegan type of egg replacer, is an excellent product for egg replacement and is available in health food stores. Ellen Degeneres's personal chef Roberto Martin recommends this type of egg replacer if you do a lot of vegan cooking. "It comes in a large container, but it's worth it," Martin says. It, too, works perfectly in any baking recipes that call for eggs.

Lactose-Free Foods

Milk replacements generally have a one-to-one ratio with milk. You can find a variety of milk replacements, including almond, rice, coconut, and hemp milks. Soy milk is also a good replacement, as long as you're not allergic to soy.

If you need to replace buttermilk, use 2 tablespoons lemon juice combined with 1 cup of a milk substitute.

 GLUTEN GAFFE

Those with a gluten intolerance may also have a sensitivity to dairy. Casein, a protein in milk, is often used as an additive in nondairy foods as well as deli meats. You may see it noted as *caseinate*. Ghee, which is clarified butter, has had all milk solids removed. Casein is not present in ghee, if it has been correctly made.

The Least You Need to Know

- Wheat flour replacements are often high in nutrients, such as amino acids, vitamins, carbs, and protein.
- Nut flours, such as almond or hazelnut, are great protein-packed replacements, as long as nut allergies aren't a concern.
- Dried beans are often milled to create flour.
- When you replace wheat flour with a substitute, you might need to include additional starches.
- Guar gum and xanthan gum are gluten-free baking additives that help bind the different flour ingredients.
- Those who are gluten intolerant may also benefit from avoiding eggs and dairy. Soy could be another troublesome ingredient.

CHAPTER 4

What Not to Eat

More than 10,000 years ago, the hunter-gatherers started planting seeds, and that led to farming. Fast-forward to today, and you'll find breads, cereals, and grain-related products in the majority of homes.

Unfortunately, a lot of those cereals, breads, and bread-based foods make us sick. Some of those products, like wheat, barley, and rye, you know for certain contain gluten. Others, like triticale, spelt, and einkorn, you might not have even heard of, let alone know about their potential gluten content.

By the end of this chapter, you'll be well versed in all the gluten-containing grains you need to avoid. You learn to identify some hidden sources of gluten, too. This chapter gives you the basic knowledge you need to interpret food labels and avoid the foods that are bad for you.

In This Chapter

- Gluten-filled grains to avoid
- Avoiding gluten in processed foods
- Tips for spotting hidden gluten
- Some foods iffy on gluten content

Wheat

Wheat is the third most-produced grain in the world, after corn and rice. The United States, Russia, and China are the biggest wheat producers. Although it's grown in most states, Kansas and North Dakota lead in U.S. wheat production. But wheat, its products, and its by-products are no good for the gluten-intolerant.

According to the Whole Grains Council, wheat became popular because it's easy to detach the wheat from the chaff, and dough made from wheat flour is wonderfully pliable and versatile. Wheat flour can be used for making everything from doughnuts and cakes, to pita bread and spaghetti.

 FOOD FOR THOUGHT

Sometimes wheat starch is used to strengthen paper during its manufacturing process and as a substitute for plastic. Wheatware (wheatware.com), for example, produces a wide variety of biodegradable, plastic-free products, including foodservice items and trash bags. These may be good for the environment, but as a gluten-intolerant person, you should avoid them.

Wheat is a grass with tens of thousands of varieties. (In comparison, rice only has several thousand varieties.) The precursor to today's wheat was known as *Triticeae* during our ancestors' times; the scientific family name for a wheat is *Triticum*. That's why you'll see *T. durum* (or *Triticum durum*) in some references to durum wheat. *T. spelta* is the spelt species of wheat.

Here are some other wheat products you might run across:

- Amulum, a thickening starch made from soaking wheat kernels in water

- Bulgur, used in tabbouleh salad

- Freekeh, a roasted green wheat

- Wheat germ, a potassium-rich element from the seed of the wheat berry

The categories of hard wheat or soft wheat indicate the amount of protein content. (Remember, gluten is the protein found in wheat.) Great for making breads, hard wheat has about 10 to 15 percent protein content, whereas soft wheat is more starchy and has up to 10 percent protein. It's better used for foods like cookies and cakes. Durum wheat, which is also known *T. durum* or semolina, is the hardest wheat.

You come into contact with wheat in breads, muffins, and other baked goods because wheat flour is so universally used. Standard pasta—spaghetti, vermicelli, elbow macaroni—is made from wheat, and wheat berries and bulgur are often served as side dishes.

> **TASTY TIDBIT**
>
> People often confuse cracked wheat and bulgur. Bulgur, often used in tabbouleh salad, is made from steamed or parboiled wheat kernels that are then dried and crushed. Cracked wheat, on the other hand, is the remains of the broken wheat. It's often eaten as a cereal or used in breads. If you're gluten intolerant, avoid both of these.

Wheat Berries

If you shop at a health food store, you might find wheat berries in the bulk section. For the gluten tolerant, wheat berries are a great nutritional food. For the gluten intolerant, they're off limits.

Wheat berries are hard wheat, so they're high in protein, amino acids, and B vitamins. Preparations of wheat berries include soaking them overnight and then cooking them in water. Sprouted wheat berries are sprouted to become wheatgrass.

Wheatgrass

You may see wheatgrass added to smoothies and other healthful concoctions. You might also see it as an ingredient in nutritional supplements.

Wheatgrass reportedly has high *antioxidant* activity. It seems a no-brainer that gluten-intolerant people should avoid anything with *wheat* in its name, but then we have buck*wheat*, which *is* gluten-free, so some people assume all other "healthful" wheat products are also gluten-free. They're not.

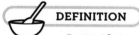

> **DEFINITION**
>
> **Antioxidants,** such as ascorbic acid found in citrus, help prevent food from oxidizing or becoming rotten. Some scientists suggest antioxidants can aid in reducing heart disease and cancer. Vitamins E and C are examples of antioxidants.

There's some debate about whether wheatgrass is safe for those with glucose intolerance. Because it's an early sprout of the wheat berry, wheatgrass is a vegetable and, therefore, has no gluten. Some producers of wheatgrass claim their wheatgrass is free of gluten because of the processes used. However, it's very important to note that cross-contamination could be rampant with wheatgrass, so to be safe, many people with gluten intolerance avoid it.

What should you do about wheatgrass? Don't just take anyone's advice on the matter. Avoid it until you've checked with your health-care professional, who should be able to give you an answer and guide you if you want to add wheatgrass to your diet.

Semolina

Milling the endosperm of durum (remember the *Triticum durum* from earlier?) creates semolina. The hardest of hard wheat, semolina is used to make pasta and couscous. Its incredibly high gluten content allows pasta dough to stretch without breaking.

If you like couscous but can no longer eat wheat products, you might consider cooking quinoa as a suitable substitute.

Barley

Barley, a wheat relative, has less gluten than wheat, but it's still on the foods-to-avoid list if you're gluten intolerant. High in fiber and antioxidants, barley has been shown to lower LDL cholesterol, the "bad" cholesterol.

Because it's a hardy grower, barley is a staple grain in many parts of the world. You might have had barley in a soup or stew or as a breakfast porridge or side dish. Barley can also be found as an ingredient in quick and yeast breads. Barley is the grain used to make many beers, so avoid all but the gluten-free varieties of beer.

Just as wheat has some by-products, barley has some, too, and you need to be wary of them.

Barley Malt

Barley malt is another reason it's important for you to understand what you read in ingredient lists. Malt is sprouted (or germinated) grain that's been dried, a process referred to as *malting*.

Barley is often the grain used for making malt, and it's used in many products, including malt flavoring, malt extract, malt syrup, malted milk, and malt vinegar. If you're shopping for a product that includes "malt" in the name, be careful that it's not malt from barley. Rice or corn malt are two alternatives.

GLUTEN GAFFE

You're shopping and pick up a wheat-free product. You read the ingredients list and find a reference to "malt extract." This should raise a red flag. If the ingredient list isn't more specific about what the extract is exactly, call the manufacturer to confirm what grain was used to make the malt extract. Remember that *wheat free* does not always mean "gluten free."

Barley Grass

Barley grass is high in antioxidants. But like wheatgrass, controversy abounds as to whether barley grass is safe for those with gluten intolerance. Because the grain is what contains the protein gluten, some claim barley grass is gluten free.

However, like wheatgrass, the possibility of cross-contamination becomes a concern. Avoid barley grass until you've discussed it with your health-care professional or a dietitian.

Rye

Rye is a grain that grows more quickly than wheat and can thrive in harsh conditions. In fact, rye was considered a weed at one point, until farmers recognized its potential. Northern Europe grows and consumes the majority of rye, although the grain may have initially arrived from central Asia.

Rye is high in fiber and antioxidants—two reasons for its popularity. While rye contains some gluten, it does not perform as well as the gluten found in wheat, which explains the heavy density of rye breads such as pumpernickel. Rye is also used to create *kvass,* a fermented drink.

FOOD FOR THOUGHT

Rye starch, used in the manufacture of some plastics and matches, can also be found in adhesives.

Oats

Oats, which are abundant in antioxidants, are highly rated for their ability to keep you full long after eating them. They've also been found to play a role in lowering bad cholesterol and blood pressure, and reduce the risk for some cancers and Type 2 diabetes.

Oats, like rye, were originally thought to be a weed. But unlike rye, oats actually do *not* contain gluten. So why are they on the do-not-eat list? Because there's a possibility that most of the oats and oat-related products you find on grocery store shelves may be cross-contaminated with glutenous grains such as wheat.

Some manufacturers source their oats from gluten-free areas and work hard to process them in a gluten-free environment. Then they test for gluten to ensure their oats aren't contaminated. (The government allows for 20 parts per million; some manufacturers test at a lower parts per million.) Bob's Red Mill, Glutenfreeda Foods, Montana Gluten Free, and Trader Joe's are a few brands that sell gluten-free oats.

If you're just beginning to avoid gluten, don't immediately eat oats. Consult with your health-care provider first. There's a chance you may need to avoid all oats, or avoid them until your lower intestinal villi have had a chance to settle into the gluten-free diet.

A good substitute in recipes that call for rolled oats is quinoa flakes.

Triticale

Triticale (*triht-ih-KAY-lee*) is a hybrid of rye and wheat. Its name comes from a combination of wheat from the *Triticum* family and rye from the *Secale* family. Developed to provide the advantages of wheat and the growing ability of rye, the triticale berry, flake, and flour are used in cooking.

Relatively speaking, triticale contains a small amount of gluten. Its flour can be used in quick breads and yeasted breads, but because of its low levels of gluten, it's often combined with wheat flour to improve elasticity.

Spelt

Spelt, also called dinkel or dinkle, is a variety of wheat, like durum wheat. You may see spelt used in quick breads, yeast breads, and pasta. Spelt is touted as easier to digest than wheat, but as a relative of wheat, it has gluten.

However, if you have a wheat insensitivity rather than celiac disease, you *might* be able to eat spelt. Unless your health-care provider or dietitian has cleared you for eating spelt, avoid it.

Kamut

Kamut is a variety of wheat that can be traced back to the time of the Egyptian pharaohs. The name of this ancient wheat is *khorasan*. The trademark Kamut signals to consumers that the

Kamut khorasan is of a particular, nonhybrid, and specific quality of unmodified ancient grain. Many manufacturers sell Kamut.

You'll see Kamut as an ingredient in pastas and cereals. Although it's a high-protein grain with an interesting back story, it's not gluten-free.

Emmer

Emmer (or farro) is a grain that was a staple for the ancient Egyptians and Romans. Emmer was phased out over centuries because it's harder to mill than wheat and other wheat varieties; the kernels need to be hulled first.

Emmer resurfaced in Italy as farro and is used today in pasta and baked goods. Due to its close relation to wheat, avoid emmer and farro.

Einkorn

Einkorn is also an ancient grain that's a low-yield wheat today. There's some question as to whether it's the same species as farro or emmer. Either way, einkorn contains gluten, so avoid it on a gluten-free diet.

In health food stores, you may see packages of einkorn pasta and einkorn wheat berries. Avoid these, too.

Hidden Gluten

Now that you know the names of all the glutenous flours and wheat variations, you can look for them on ingredient lists. But what about hidden gluten? Whether from wheat or other sources, gluten is found in many packaged and processed goods, including personal-care products. Therefore, learning to spot hidden gluten is essential.

Gluten may not always be easy to spot because it often goes by unfamiliar names. For example, dextrin is an additive that's often made from wheat. Fortunately, labels can help you. Products that contain wheat derivatives are required to be labeled as containing wheat. You might see wheat in the list of ingredients or in a "contains" line at the end of the ingredients list.

 FOOD FOR THOUGHT

The 2004 Food Allergen Labeling and Consumer Protection Act (FALCPA) requires food manufacturers to label products if they contain wheat or a wheat derivative. In August 2013, the U.S. government established a standard for gluten-free labeling. Products labeled "gluten free" must fall under the 20 parts-per-million mark.

A food's label should clearly state if wheat is an ingredient. Look for gluten on the label of these processed foods:

- Milk and yogurt with flavorings

- Lunchmeats

- Salad dressings

- Shredded packaged cheese—may use flour to prevent caking

- Packaged or processed fruits and veggies, such as dried fruits or vegetables with sauces

- Soy sauce

- Cake icing

- Beef, vegetable, fish, and chicken bouillon

- Miso—may contain barley

- Some vegetarian and vegan mock meat products, such as veggie burgers

- Mock seafood, such as imitation crab

- Candy and chocolates—often barley or wheat are used as fillers

- Ice cream—some manufacturers may use oatmeal as a filler

- Wine coolers

- Lip glosses and lipstick—some use glutenous fillers

Sometimes food labels indicate that the product was manufactured at a facility that also processes wheat products. If you decide to eat such foods, be aware of any possible reactions you have.

And remember, wheat isn't the only ingredient that contains gluten. Laws are on the books now for manufacturers to label wheat-containing foods as such, but at some point, the law may change to include a requirement for labeling derivatives of rye and barley. So for now, proceed with caution.

 TASTY TIDBIT

Always check food labels, even if the product doesn't seem like the kind of food that might contain gluten. Make a note of any hidden gluten foods you find and strike them off your shopping list. And then find a safer alternative.

Does It Contain Gluten ... or Not?

Certain foods, especially pickles and blue cheese, are iffy on whether they're foods the gluten-intolerant should eat. Grain alcohols are also a concern. Let's investigate these foods a bit more so you can make an informed decision.

Pickles

Pickles are often made with vinegar, and sometimes malt vinegar is used. You know malt vinegar is made from barley. Therefore, some gluten-sensitive folks believe pickles should be avoided unless you're absolutely certain of what vinegar was used in the pickling method.

Some gluten-intolerant folks can eat pickles without any issues. In any case, you tread cautiously. Check labels, and ask your dietitian. He or she might be able to direct you further.

Blue Cheese

Blue cheese is another iffy food for those with gluten sensitivities. Why? Because the mold that gives blue cheese its distinctive hue was traditionally cultivated on pieces of bread.

Today, however, most cultures for cheese are produced in laboratories without the use of grains. *Most.* Some cheese-makers still go the more traditional route, and that's where the problem is introduced.

If you're concerned, research individual cheese-makers to learn how they get their molds and then only eat the cheese from those manufacturers that don't use bread. BelGioiso, Rogue Creamery, and Monteforte are three cheese-makers that certify their blue cheese is gluten free.

 FOOD FOR THOUGHT

The Canadian Celiac Association (CCA) did a study testing the gluten levels of five blue cheeses—three made with cultures harvested from bread, and two made with cultures grown in a laboratory. None of the cheeses, including the three traditionally made cheeses, were found to contain detectable levels of gluten. Based on these findings, the new CCA publication *Acceptability of Food and Food Ingredients for the Gluten-Free Diet* lists blue cheese as an acceptable food.

It's up to you whether blue cheese is a food you want to eat. If you do, approach it cautiously. If you have any reactions, you may want to purchase only clearly marked gluten-free blue cheese.

Regardless of your decision on the cheese itself, be wary of blue cheese dressing, which may contain glutenous additives.

Grain-Based Spirits

Many distilled spirits are made from grains that contain gluten. Whiskey may be made with barley, wheat, rye, or corn. Gin can be derived from a variety of sources but is often made using a grain. Vodka, traditionally made from potatoes, may be distilled from grain sources as well. What does this mean for the gluten intolerant person who wants to imbibe?

In theory, distilling removes the gluten, which means distilled alcohol should be okay. However, some distillers add mash, a mixture of milled grain and water, during the final stages of production, which is where gluten may be reintroduced. If you have a question, call the manufacturer and ask about the company's process. If they add mash, ask what grain the mash is made from.

How can you tell if you're having a reaction to gluten? Some folks report having a harsh hangover that doesn't correlate to the amount of alcohol consumed.

TASTY TIDBIT

A number of alcoholic beverages are acceptable for those with gluten intolerance. Consider these grain-free options: wines, including champagne and other grape-based drinks; rum, which is made from sugar cane; vodka, made from potatoes; tequila, which is made from the agave plant; and gin, made from potatoes.

You don't need to be a party pooper, but do avoid alcohols or mixers that add colors, flavors, or additives. This may be where gluten could re-enter into a supposedly gluten-free product. If you do use mixers, read the labels to be sure they're gluten free.

The Least You Need to Know

- Wheat and its cousins—barley, rye, triticale, spelt (or dinkel), Kamut, emmer (or farro), and einkorn—contain gluten and should be avoided in a gluten-free diet.
- Although oats don't contain gluten, there's a high risk of cross-contamination when oats are grown and processed.
- In addition to its inclusion in baked goods, barley is often used as a basis for malted products. Check the ingredients list before consuming.

- Although spelt (or dinkel) is an easy-to-digest relative to wheat, it still contains gluten. Your health-care provider can advise you on whether to include spelt in your diet or not.

- Read ingredient lists carefully, and be aware that although products that contain wheat require a label, products that contain barley, rye, and other grains don't.

Your Gluten-Free Kitchen

To go gluten-free, you need to eliminate all glutenous ingredients, foods, and other products from your kitchen. It can be a daunting task, but you're up to the challenge! You might find it helpful to enlist the assistance of friends and family as you purge the gluten and clean food preparation areas from previous gluten encounters.

In this chapter, we share ideas on how to approach your kitchen, remove the glutenous products, and replace them with gluten-free items. Think of it as a spring-cleaning for your kitchen—and your health. Once you've cleared out and cleaned your pantry, you can fill it with delicious, nutritious go-to gluten-free food.

Are you in a gluten-free household, or will you be negotiating shelf space with those who can eat gluten? Either way, we give you tips and precautions for staying safe in your own kitchen.

In This Chapter

- Cleaning out your pantry
- Gluten-free foods to have on hand
- Sharing a kitchen with gluten eaters
- Tips for keeping your kitchen safe

Ridding Your Pantry of Gluten

One of the first things Elizabeth did when she went gluten free was to clear her cupboards of any items that contained gluten. She started by comparing a list of ingredients she couldn't eat to the ingredient lists on items in her cupboard. What foods she could eat went back in. What she couldn't eat was set aside to be used by other family members when Elizabeth wasn't around.

Initially, Elizabeth thought she would be the only one in her family of five to eat gluten free. But within months, her husband and kids had given up gluten, too. This might happen in your household, but don't worry if it doesn't. Even if you're the only one going gluten free, you can still enjoy family mealtimes.

Clearing the Shelves

Before you rid your pantry and refrigerator of glutenous foods, take time to shop for some go-to gluten-free items. Refer to Chapter 7 for ideas, and get what you need for a few gluten-free meals. That way, when you begin purging, you'll have food on hand you can eat.

As you clear your shelves and fridge, start building your list of gluten-free replacements.

When your pantry is clear, make a meal plan and begin stocking up on gluten-free foods. Start by planning for a day or two, or even a week, and shop for only those items on your list. Straying from your list provides an opening for you to revert to buying other products that aren't as good for your health.

 TASTY TIDBIT

Remember, you're not just checking labels to get *rid* of food; you're also learning what you can *keep*. Even though the packaging might not have a special gluten-free indicator, check the ingredients anyway. Many food manufacturers that produce gluten-free goods haven't yet started using their packaging to highlight their gluten-free status.

Plans for Your Excess Food

If you live in a house with others who can still consume gluten, ask them to use any remaining glutenous products you've culled from the pantry. If having glutenous products in the house proves to be too tempting, consider donating the food. Some places might not take such foods, but it doesn't hurt to ask, and your gluten purge could help out a local food bank. If not, maybe friends and family would want the glutenous food.

While you're passing off the semolina pasta to your sister-in-law, co-worker, or neighbor, speak with them about your new diet. Talking to friends and family about what you can't eat gives them an opportunity to ask questions and understand why it's so important for you to avoid gluten. And handing over food you can't eat is one way to introduce the subject of your gluten-free journey, one way to start the conversation.

Shedding the Gluten

When you're taking on your cabinets and shelves, get rid of these items that contain gluten:

- Breads and pastries
- Flours (wheat, rye, barley, and oat)
- Pastas
- Cereals (hot and cold)
- Bread and cake mixes
- Couscous
- Flavored rice mixes
- Malt vinegar

Check the labels of these items for the possibility of gluten:

- Barbecue sauces
- Cornmeal (check to be sure it's not mixed with wheat flour)
- Frozen processed foods
- Salad dressings
- Soy sauce
- Flavored salts
- Condiments (some mustards and ketchups may contain gluten)

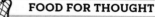 **FOOD FOR THOUGHT**

Even though they're used as additives, MSG and autolyzed yeast extract are gluten free.

If you see any of these ingredients on labels, put the food in the purge pile:

- Wheat and anything with wheat in its name, like hydrolyzed wheat gluten or wheat germ

- Barley

- Oats

- Rye

- Spelt

- Graham flour

- Enriched flour

- Cookie dough or cookie crumbs

Avoid the Additives

Celiac and gluten-intolerant people eat whole foods for many reasons, but avoiding *additives* is one of the primary ones.

> **DEFINITION**
>
> An **additive** is a substance food manufacturers incorporate into the production of various food items. With around 3,000 additives available, they're used in numerous ways, including increasing nutrition, helping preserve foods, or making the food taste better.

The additives in prepackaged foods may or may not contain gluten. Artificial colors, dextrins, emulsifiers, glucose syrup, and food starch are just a few ingredients often made with wheat or wheat by-products. Caramel color, if it's made with barley malt or starch hydrolysates made with wheat, could also contain gluten.

You may receive mixed answers about additives because of where the foods are produced. For example, in the United States, caramel color may be okay. When it's from other countries, probably not. When in doubt, call the food's manufacturer and ask. Skip the food until you've confirmed it's gluten free.

Stop Cross-Contamination

You also need to dispose of foods that may have been contaminated by gluten. For example, jam, butter, and other spreads are easily contaminated by breadcrumbs if someone scoops them from the jar with the same knife they used for spreading them on bread.

If your household operates like this, you'll need to enforce a new set of rules. You could use a spoon to remove the product and then spread it with a knife. This way, the spoon doesn't touch the bread and the knife doesn't touch the spread.

Avoid any foods you fear may have been contaminated. If someone within your home can still eat the jelly, for instance, mark the jar to remind yourself it's not safe for you to eat.

If your home is completely gluten free, donate the contaminated items to friends or family. Or if you have no other option, throw them away.

Clean, Conquer, Reorganize?

When you empty your kitchen of gluten-containing goods, take some time to clean and reorganize it. You might find that eating gluten free means eating at home more often, so take the time to put things where they better serve you in your kitchen.

A friend of Elizabeth's has placed stations around her kitchen where certain activities take place. For example, you might have a station for your bread maker, if you choose to make your own bread. Having stations can help contain any potential gluten contamination. But being organized will certainly make you feel more comfortable in your kitchen—and more willing to make the effort to cook gluten-free meals.

You could also clear space in the freezer or refrigerator for various flours. Almond flour, xanthan gum, and other products keep better if you freeze them. Elizabeth keeps many of her flours in alphabetical order inside her freezer door, which makes them easy to locate.

 FOOD FOR THOUGHT

You can store many gluten-free flours in airtight containers in your pantry up to 6 months. For longer usage, store them in the freezer.

Stocking Your Gluten-Free Kitchen

When re-stocking your pantry after you've purged it of glutenous products, start by replacing the items you use most often. Consider what you eat during a regular week and what staples you like to have on hand, and add those first.

If you're accustomed to making a quick meal of pasta and vegetables when you're short on time, what will happen if you remove those boxes of spaghetti you relied on without replacing them with a gluten-free substitute? Think about your eating habits, and plan ahead.

Whole Foods

When it comes to must-have ingredients, start with whole foods. This includes unprocessed meats, fresh vegetables, and whole grains. Think about choosing foods that are as close to their natural state as possible. The closer you can get to eating food that's not processed, the less chance you have of ingesting gluten.

Michael Pollan's book *Food Rules: An Eater's Manual* provides tips on eating more healthfully. One of our favorites that may help you is to try to picture the foods you're purchasing in their natural states. For example, cheese crackers may taste yummy, but have you ever seen a cheese cracker tree or plant?

Whole foods are rich in nutrients, and they're a great way to make up for the nutrients you may be missing because of your gluten intolerance. Vegetables, fruits, meats, eggs, and dairy (without malt flavorings) are all gluten free. If you add other ingredients as you cook these foods, be sure the additional ingredients are free of gluten as well.

Organic and Local Foods

Also consider eating fruits and vegetables that are organic or locally sourced. Most fruits and vegetables begin losing nutrients as soon as they're harvested, so the longer it takes for these foods to reach your plate, the fewer nutrients you receive. Buying fresh and local foods can help ensure your body receives the freshest, richest nutrients possible.

Other great things happen when you start buying local foods. You start to meet people who grow your foods, and you also meet like-minded people in your community. (More about that in Chapter 12.) But the main benefit to shopping locally is that the foods you buy and eat tend to taste better, and if you can talk directly to the farmer, you can learn how he or she is raising the chickens and whose eggs you're making into omelets.

Coops and CSAs

Elizabeth's town features a cooperative of area farmers who deliver their fresh ingredients to several locations around town. She can get online, order by noon Wednesday, and have her groceries delivered to a convenient location on Thursday. The meats and vegetables are always fresh, and she knows she's helping out a local farmer.

If you don't have such a service, maybe a cooperative in your area specializes in local products. Some food coops are actual grocery stores—that's where Jeanette does most of her shopping—but others are simply organized groups of people who pool their resources for good prices.

Some food cooperatives also organize a *CSA* or *community supported agriculture,* which can provide you with local produce. Both Elizabeth and Jeanette have enjoyed the benefits of joining CSAs. As CSA members, they give their respective farmers seed money, and every week during the growing season, they each receive a large box of fresh vegetables and fruits. These programs can help sustain whole foods and farmers in your area.

DEFINITION

CSA is the acronym for **community supported agriculture.** In many communities, farmers sell shares of, or a subscription to, their crops to a limited number of people. Most operate by charging a lump sum before spring planting. Then, at regular intervals during the growing season, customers pick up the fresh farm foods from a central location or pay to have it delivered to their homes. Many food cooperatives and health food stores help promote such programs.

Farmers' Markets

Many communities also have farmers' markets where you can go, meet the farmers, and buy directly from them. Farmers' markets are great communal events, and some even feature live music. Where else can you find fresh food and community?

Beware of the stands selling baked goods at farmers' markets. Unless you can speak directly to the baker, you won't know for sure what products were used when making the baked goods. Some may sell gluten-free products, but many feature gluten-based products.

When you get to know people, such as the farmers and bakers, they start to get to know you, too, and they can learn about your gluten-free needs. Friendliness can help you build rapport with the sales people, which helps them remember you and your gluten intolerance.

But remember, you're becoming a gluten-free expert in your own right, so always read labels. As friendly as everyone may be, and as helpful as they might be, you are your own advocate, and you need to ensure you're eating the right things.

Other Gluten-Free Grocery Items

Bread, one of the major staples you may miss, is a subject that you'll get a *lot* of opinions about (and many from those who aren't gluten free). If you want to start buying gluten-free bread, be sure it's made in a gluten-free facility. You don't want cross-contamination to ruin your first slice. Some of Elizabeth's favorites are the different varieties of Rudi's, Udi's, and Sami's Bakery breads. She's found that many gluten-free breads do better if you keep them in the freezer and toast them as you need them.

Do you bake? If not, you might want to consider giving it a try. When you start, you'll want to think about what flours you'd like to try and invest in a few. Sweet rice, white rice, and brown rice flours are good to have on hand for making sandwich bread. Almond flour has a rich taste and can be used to make yummy breakfast treats. For beginning bakers, gluten-free flour blends are also good to have on hand to make pancakes or cookies. Although these flours can be more expensive than wheat flour, buying flours to make your own breads is less expensive than buying manufactured bread. Bob's Red Mill, King Arthur Flour, and even Trader Joe's make gluten-free flour blends.

Familiar grains are a go-to item for many with gluten intolerance. Stock up on gluten-free rice and polenta. Can't eat corn? Experiment with quinoa. Do you eat a lot of pasta? Try some of the many gluten-free pastas on the market. Many are made with rice, but you'll find varieties made with quinoa, buckwheat, sweet potato, and other ingredients. Explore the different flavors and textures offered.

Replace gluten-filled condiments with ones that aren't manufactured or contaminated with gluten. Invest in some gluten-free broths and salad dressings—or make your own. (See Chapter 14 for some delicious and easy recipes.) Regular soy sauce contains gluten, so look to San-J brand Tamari and Bragg Liquid Aminos as good soy sauce replacements.

> **GLUTEN GAFFE**
>
> Condiments can frequently be an afterthought in food preparation. A hamburger without a bun is gluten free ... until you've added the mustard that contains gluten. Be careful when considering what condiments to keep.

Eating nutrient-rich foods doesn't mean you can't also enjoy foods like pizza every now and then. More and more gluten-free options are available in the frozen food section, and these can be great to have on hand for nights when you don't have time or energy to cook. Take time to explore the gluten-free frozen pizzas available and find one you like. Just remember to balance these meals with less-processed foods.

No matter if you're gluten free or not, snacking happens. Be sure you have some gluten-free crackers or bread available. The marketplace is also bursting with other gluten-free snacks like potato chips and popcorn.

Kitchen Equipment

Clean, gluten-free kitchen equipment is a must when you're eating gluten free. All the gluten-free breads and ingredients in the world won't make a difference to your health if they're regularly contaminated by your kitchen tools and equipment.

You may need to invest in some new kitchen equipment, especially if you're the only one in your household who's gluten free. If you prepare most of the family meals, you also might want to have a family meeting to explain the parameters of your new gluten-free kitchen zone.

You might want to have duplicates of some items, especially those that tend to come in close contact with gluten. For example, if you have a roommate who makes a lot of chocolate-chip cookies with wheat flour, purchase your own spatula and keep it in a container with other utensils marked "Gluten Free." Or mark a big "GF" on the handle with a marker.

Instead of buying additional baking sheets, you could use aluminum foil or parchment paper between your baked goods and the baking sheet to avoid potential contamination.

 TASTY TIDBIT

A well-stocked kitchen includes pots and pans of various sizes. (Elizabeth's medium saucepan gets a daily workout!) In certain homes—with some individuals eating gluten and others not—you might need to have duplicate items or deal with potential cross-contamination.

Here's a list of some kitchen equipment you might want to upgrade to or buy if you don't already have them:

Food processor   A food processor or, if you can afford it, a Vitamix, is useful for all sorts of dishes. Elizabeth uses her food processor for everything from making gluten-free date bars to her own almond flour.

Good knives   No doubt, good knives can be expensive. But they're well worth the investment. An 8-inch chef's knife is a good knife to start with. If a knife has been used to cut something with gluten, be sure to clean it with soap and hot water. It's also important to have a knife steel to sharpen your knife blades.

Spatulas and wooden spoons   You may already have a collection of spatulas and wooden spoons. If you're living in a divided household with some inhabitants eating gluten items, mark and segregate your gluten-free cooking utensils.

Mixing bowls   A set of nested glass mixing bowls works for many types of food preparation, from stirring cake batter to tossing salads. Look for a set with rubber lids so you can use the bowls to save leftovers, too.

Electric mixer   An electric mixer, either a stand mixer or a handheld version, is great for whipping up gluten-free breads and cakes.

Colander   If you've ever strained your cooked pasta, you probably know residual starch remains on the colander. Consider purchasing a duplicate colander if you have gluten-containing foods in your kitchen.

Bread maker Gluten-free breads can be expensive, and making homemade bread by hand is time-consuming. Investing in a bread maker can save you time and money if you use it regularly. Be careful if others in the household want to use it because cross-contamination will occur if others use wheat, rye, barley, or oat flours in their bread.

Avoiding Gluten in a Gluten Household

If someone in the household prepares foods with gluten, take the time to clean where the preparation appeared. Obviously, they can clean up as well, but you might feel more security if you take charge of the cleanup.

Use hot, soapy water for general cleanup, and a stronger-cleaning spray for deeper cleaning. Disinfectant wipes also come in handy.

Create Gluten-Free Zones

If you're the only gluten-intolerant eater in the house, keep your foods and kitchen equipment separate from your gluten-eating cohabitants. Nothing sends a clearer message that your gluten-free foods are important, and that this division needs to be respected. Segregating your foods also enables you to immediately see when and if you need to replenish your gluten-free items.

In addition to establishing gluten-free space in the fridge and cabinets, you might want to designate certain prep areas as your gluten-free workspaces. Stake your claim on sections of the counter and table or specific cutting boards.

Get Separate Equipment

If those you live with aren't interested in going gluten free, or if you suspect they may not be willing to follow your guidelines to avoid contamination, consider having duplicates of commonly used items in addition to those already mentioned. This includes utensils and appliances that might come in contact with gluten, such as knives and toasters, as well as products that may be contaminated, such as jam and cheese. Be sure to clearly label your set as gluten free. When you have visitors, be sure they know which utensils and appliances they can use with gluten and which cannot come in contact with it.

If you're the only one in the house who's gluten intolerant, you must take precautions. If you're not sure if something is clean, clean it again. This goes for cabinets, counters, spoons, knives, and anything else you suspect has come in contact with gluten.

TASTY TIDBIT

Contamination can happen quickly, so get into a habit of washing (by hand, if necessary) before you use something.

Kitchen Tips

As you prepare your own gluten-free meals, you may find that cooking at home is less expensive—and safer—than eating out. However, this can be daunting, especially for those who are used to grabbing prepared foods or going out to eat.

If you're not confident in the kitchen, taking some cooking classes will definitely ease your anxieties about food preparation. Basic classes like knife skills and making stock should be naturally gluten free, but call ahead and explain to the instructor your needs.

Some cooking classes are just demonstration, and it won't matter if they're gluten free or not. You can learn by observation, and you don't have to taste the food. But others involve participation, and those are some of the most fun.

If time and scheduling don't allow you to actually go to a cooking class, the internet can come to your rescue. YouTube (youtube.com) is a great resource for everything from sharpening a knife to making red velvet cake.

Many cooking experts also include mini lessons on their websites. Culinary memoirist Kathleen Flinn offers a free knife skills online cooking class at her website, kathleenflinn.com.

You can even find gluten-free cooking classes. Restaurants, cooking schools, and even community centers offer classes, and some have gluten-free classes. Glutenfreeda offers all sorts of gluten-free information, including video demonstrations of gluten-free recipes at its website (glutenfreeda.com).

Best Practices

Preparing your kitchen for gluten-free cooking takes a bit of time and money, but it's well worth the investment. But even as you can take comfort that your home can be a safe place to eat, you still may want to wipe down surfaces before you start cooking.

This is especially true if friends and family who eat gluten visit or live with you. If someone brings food into your home, ask questions and, if possible, read the labels before the products are even out of their bags.

Whenever someone brings gluten-containing food into your home, be sure it doesn't cross-contaminate surfaces or utensils. Point out the gluten-free zones you've established. If the area does become contaminated, clean the surface well using soapy, hot water.

Consider being hyper-vigilant, especially in the beginning. Once friends and family see how serious your need is for gluten-free zones, the easier it will be for them to support you in your quest for a safe, gluten-free kitchen.

The Least You Need to Know

- Take the time to buy a few gluten-free foods before cleaning out your kitchen, so you won't be tempted to eat the food that's bad for you.
- Remove any tempting gluten-filled foods that might encourage you to cheat, and replace them with gluten-free versions.
- Additives and condiments may be a source of hidden gluten. When in doubt, throw it out (or at least don't eat it).
- Organize your kitchen so you can easily tell if you're running out of a gluten-free staple.
- If you're the only one in your home who's gluten free, take some time to explain your new dietary restrictions to your housemates.
- Label utensils to indicate if they're to be used only for gluten-free cooking, and keep them separate from utensils used for cooking gluten items.

CHAPTER 6

Gluten-Free Grocery Shopping

Grocery shopping has gotten easier for gluten-free eaters in recent years. Gluten-free products are now regularly available on the shelves at most major chain grocery stores, and food packaging is better than ever at highlighting which products are free of gluten. You may not find everything you need at the major grocery store chains where you regularly shop, but you've got plenty of options.

In this chapter, we help you figure out what you can put in your shopping cart, and we give you tips for navigating the grocery store, health food stores, and specialty food stores. The internet is also a big help in terms of getting gluten-free goods, especially if you don't have choices in your local brick-and-mortar stores. You might find yourself setting a new schedule of weekly shopping, or you might find it easier to buy items in bulk. We discuss both options in this chapter.

We also take a look at food labels in this chapter so you can identify those ingredients that are okay for you to eat. We're even going to review some packaged gluten-free foods that might help make your gluten-free transition easier. Finally, we take a look at naturally gluten-free foods. You might be surprised at the foods available for your gluten-free table!

In This Chapter

- Where to find gluten-free foods
- Understanding food labels
- Shopping for packaged gluten-free foods
- Foods naturally free of gluten

Where to Shop

Maybe you've heard that when food shopping, you should stay along the perimeter of the super-market. We think this is good advice, too. Look at your local grocery store and notice how it's laid out. Generally, the whole foods that are healthier—and safer for you to eat—are located along the walls of every grocery store. So if you shop along the walls, you'll be browsing the whole foods. Generally, the aisles in the middle of the store contain more processed foods.

 FOOD FOR THOUGHT

> In your town, you may have more flexibility in health food stores—or no flexibility. Planning for grocery shopping is a key element in eating gluten free. Make a list and then plan how to get your gluten-free shopping done. You may find that some stores accommodate your gluten intolerance more than others, and you can build your shopping plans around those stores.

What does this have to do with gluten-free shopping? The more you avoid the processed foods, the more easily you avoid the gluten lurking in such manufactured foods. There's not one bit of gluten in a bunch of carrots or a head of broccoli. Nor is there gluten in a plain, fresh chicken breast or lamb chop.

Buying unprocessed foods is one of the best things you can do for your gluten intolerance. Besides avoiding gluten, you're doing well for the other parts of your body. Before your diagnosis, you might have grabbed the precooked meat with gravy and a side of veggies that you found in your grocer's deli after work. That meal—as easy as it is to assemble and reheat—not only contains hidden gluten, but it also is packed with sodium, sugar, and fat. It also most likely contains preservatives and additives to give it a longer shelf life and make it taste better. Processed is never as high quality as fresh.

When you buy uncooked chicken breasts, vegetables, and potatoes to make your own meal, you control the amount of fat, sodium, and sugar that ends up in the finished dish. You also don't add any preservatives or additives—things your body doesn't need! By going gluten free and cooking more meals from scratch, you and your loved ones will naturally eat more healthfully.

Now, although the majority of the food items along the perimeter of grocery stores are naturally safe and gluten-free, you still have to beware of hidden culprits. Those chicken breasts marinated in teriyaki sauce? They have gluten. That ranch dressing in the ready-made salad? Glutenous. That presliced turkey meat? Most likely contaminated with gluten. With any prepackaged and already prepared food items, read labels and talk to grocery clerks to be sure it's safe for you to eat.

Grocery Stores

Take a walk through your grocery store, and you'll see that gluten-free food choices have expanded in recent years. Elizabeth's neighborhood chain grocery store has even started labeling gluten-free foods on the shelves. These can be helpful, but don't rely on them too heavily. Look for government-regulated labels (more on these later in this chapter).

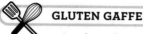 **GLUTEN GAFFE**

> Anything that contains wheat contains gluten, but if a product is labeled "wheat free" it doesn't necessarily mean it's gluten free. Remember, gluten appears in other grains.

Before you start gluten-free shopping, it helps to make a list. Then, when you're at the store, don't stray from your list. If you're looking for a brand of gluten-free deli cheese and the store appears to be out, don't settle for just any cheese. In fact, ask one of the clerks or visit the customer service desk. Yes, that may take time, but think about how your request for a gluten-free item can expand the knowledge of the store personnel. It also helps you get to know the clerks, and the more you know who's preparing and stocking your foods, the better the connection you have to your food.

When you speak with someone in a polite, calm manner, they'll more likely help you find either a substitute for your preferred item, or they might even locate stock for you that hasn't yet made it to the grocery store floor. Some managers will even order the food for you if it's not an item the store usually carries. The grocery store clerk and customer service manager do not want to lose their clientele. If you have a difficult experience, let the corporate office know about it.

Depending on where you live, you could try some of the chain grocers making gluten-free more easily accessible, including Trader Joe's, Whole Foods, Harris Teeter, Stop and Shop, Walmart, or Wegmans. Elizabeth has found many gluten-free foods and other items at Costco. Many of the gluten-free products are well labeled, but you won't find aisles devoted to gluten-free food. And the folks providing samples don't always have the correct nutritional information, so always check the labels of any food before you taste it in the store.

Health Food Stores

Health food stores are a great source for gluten-free items. As with regular grocery stores, shopping the perimeter still applies. Look for the least-processed goods along the outside of the store. In addition to finding great meats and veggies, health food stores often stock gluten-free flours in bulk, which can be cost-efficient.

At a health food store or cooperative store, you might have an easier time finding some of the new-to-you flours and specialty gluten-free items. Of the two health food stores in Elizabeth's city, one consistently stocks sweet rice flour, and the other stocks the pizza crusts Elizabeth's kids like.

Health food stores are accustomed to handling food intolerance questions because in many cases, they've catered to such customers for years. They may also be the best source for certain vitamins and supplements.

Besides just browsing the aisles, don't be afraid to pick up a phone and call the store in advance. If you see an unfamiliar ingredient in a new recipe you want to try, call and ask if it's something the store carries. It may take some time to figure out which stores carry certain products, and you might not be able to rely on one-stop shopping. However, you'll almost certainly discover new favorite foods to enjoy.

Gluten sensitivities should be a consideration when you're buying items prepared in any store, even health food stores. Do you know if the deli clerk cleaned the knife after spreading the mayonnaise? Did the clerk clean the cutting board between cutting the dinner rolls and slicing the pineapple? If you're not sure, ask. Don't risk buying the prepared-in-store foods that might have been unknowingly contaminated.

Gluten-Free and Specialty Stores

Specialty stores are cropping up in communities across the United States. Gluten-free bakeries, cupcake stores featuring a daily flavor of gluten-free cupcake, and cafés that specialize in providing gluten-free options are all growing enterprises. Some of them even update their Facebook pages with daily specials to entice gluten-free customers to stop by.

For example, in her Milwaukee neighborhood, Jeanette often shops at a store called Gluten-Free Trading Post. It's the only place where she can find gluten-free *panko* breadcrumbs.

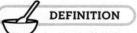 **DEFINITION**

> **Panko** are large, coarse style of breadcrumbs. They're a specialty type of breadcrumbs, often used in Japanese cuisine. You can use them in recipes that call for regular breadcrumbs.

Ethnic food markets, such as Asian and Italian markets, also stock many gluten-free options. Elizabeth has purchased *besan* (or chickpea) flour, which is a used in Indian cuisine, from her local Asian market. Jeanette has also found tapioca and rice-flour spring roll wraps at such stores. Read the labels carefully when purchasing, and ask the clerks.

On the Web

The internet makes gluten-free shopping nearly hassle free. Amazon.com can provide some general gluten-free goods, and specialty websites are devoted to gluten-free eating, making it easy to locate and purchase gluten-free foods and other items. You might even find some new gluten-free delights, too.

Lots of good gluten-free stores and websites are online. Here are a few we like that specialize in health foods or gluten-free foods:

- The Gluten-Free Mall (celiac.com/glutenfreemall) is *the* specialty gluten-free shop website. It offers a wide selection and often runs sales.

- Gluten Free $save (glutenfreesaver.com) offers daily deals. It's a fun way to try new products.

- Vitacost (vitacost.com) is where Elizabeth started ordering supplements. The day the shop held a sale on gluten-free foods, she was hooked!

- iHerb.com (iherb.com) stocks gluten-free goods and supplements.

When ordering online, be sure you're ordering gluten-free items. Some manufacturers produce a gluten-filled and a gluten-free version of the same product, so double- and triple-check the ingredient lists so you don't order the wrong one.

Reading Food Labels

Before you determined gluten was off-limits, you may never have noticed the list of allergens on a food label. Now it's time to familiarize yourself with the labels and what they mean.

Labels, Your Allergy, and Government Regulations

The good news is that the U.S. government regulates the information food manufacturers must label on their products. The bad news is that the laws are a bit hazy when it comes to gluten.

It might seem daunting at first, but once you know how to read labels and what words to look for, gluten-free shopping becomes easier, and you'll be able to detect hidden gluten in no time.

The U.S. government regulates the information food manufacturers are required to put on processed foods. If you have an allergy, you might have heard of the Food Allergen Labeling and Consumer Protection Act of 2004 (FALCPA). This legislation lays out the food allergy labeling guidelines for eight major allergens: milk, egg, fish, crustacean shellfish, tree nuts, peanuts, soybeans, and wheat. With this list, the Food and Drug Administration (FDA) issues rules for food manufacturers to follow when labeling their products to let buyers know about potential allergens in the ingredients.

 TASTY TIDBIT

The FDA shares a list of naturally gluten-free options, such as milk *not* flavored with malt and other gluten-containing ingredients, on its website. No brand-name products are given, but the site does offer a lot of foods that don't contain gluten, including fresh fruits and vegetables, butter and eggs, tree nuts and peanuts, fresh fish and shellfish, and "non-gluten-containing grains, such as corn." Visit fda.gov/ForConsumers/ConsumerUpdates/ucm265212.htm.

Are There Gluten Standards?

In August 2013, the FDA issued a final rule for the voluntary labeling of gluten-free foods by August 2014. Food manufacturers may claim a food or a dietary supplement is gluten free if it doesn't contain wheat, barley, or rye. (The FDA suggests cross-contamination of oats is preventable and does not include oats in this listing.)

However, foods can also claim a gluten-free label if they contain wheat, barley, or rye *and* are processed to remove gluten to contain less than 20 parts per million (ppm). One example of this is wheat starch. According to the National Foundation for Celiac Awareness, if a 1-ounce piece of bread contains less than 20 ppm, there would be less than 1 milligram gluten.

The FDA's gluten-free regulations do not impact alcohol, alcoholic beverages, prescription and over-the-counter drugs, makeup, and U.S. Department of Agriculture foods. It does align the gluten-free labeling in the United States more closely with Europe, Canada, and other international standards.

To protect yourself, always read labels carefully and watch out for inconsistent or, in some cases, nonexistent labeling. Remember, gluten hazards—such as prepackaged foods that don't call out the ingredients in glutenous soy sauce or deli meat without a readily available ingredients list—still lurk in the grocery store.

In addition, some grains ordinarily considered safe, such as oats, sometimes have tested positive for gluten. Often foods become cross-contaminated because of proximity of the grain to wheat or other glutenous crops during the growing and/or processing phase.

So if you or someone in your house is a gluten-free eater, you must read labels vigilantly and be knowledgeable about different ingredients that could pose potential problems.

Know Your Ingredients

Reading labels is one thing. Understanding what you're reading is another. You need to be able to interpret what you read, keeping in mind how you react to specific ingredients. As you grow more accustomed to gluten-free eating, your body may have more pronounced reactions to certain foods. This is probably your body letting you know a food contains gluten. This might even happen with foods that didn't cause reactions before.

Keeping a food journal is helpful in cases like this. In your journal, list specific brands along with your reactions to them. After reviewing your journal, you'll better know which brands to reach for when you shop and which ones to avoid.

Unfortunately, you may still suffer some unpleasant surprises. For example, you always purchase your favorite honey mustard salad dressing, but once, after eating your dinner salad, you feel sick. What happened? It's entirely possible the food manufacturer changed its formula for the dressing, and it now contains gluten. *Always* read labels when shopping, even for your familiar favorites.

 GLUTEN GAFFE

> Food manufacturers often change their recipes or formulas without warning consumers. Always read labels of packaged and processed foods, even if certain products never bothered you in the past.

What to Avoid

If all you needed to do to eat gluten free was to avoid wheat, your task would be easier. But other grains contain gluten, too. Rye, triticale, barley, and spelt all contain gluten, even if they're not technically wheat. The Celiac Sprue Association (csaceliacs.info) suggests using the acronym *WBRO* for remembering what substances to avoid. *WBRO* stands for "wheat, barley, rye, and oats."

If a product is made with flour, it's most likely made with wheat. Standard crackers, cookies, bagels, breads, pastas, and cereals are made with wheat and pose a problem for those avoiding gluten.

Remember, too, that wheat is used as a thickener for many sauces and gravies. Even dairy products, sauces, and processed meats may use wheat or wheat-derivative fillers, such as the modified food starch mentioned earlier.

Wheat comes in a variety of forms and products. What about products that aren't the "standard" wheat foods? If you're looking to vary your diet, you might be interested in nonbakery items such as pasta. But be careful. These items might contain wheat that goes by a different, less-common name, such as Kamut or khorasan wheat.

It's important to understand where else gluten appears. For example, is there gluten in couscous or farina? What about seitan or wheat germ? Yes. These products *always* contain wheat. If the product is produced in another country, the labeling might not specifically mention wheat as an ingredient, but it's there.

Some products contain disguised versions of wheat. When labels include vegetable protein or *modified food starch,* be aware that these can be made with wheat. Barley, a gluten-containing ingredient, can also be used in *natural flavorings.*

> **DEFINITION**
>
> A **modified food starch** is a starch that's altered in some way—sometimes even using chemicals. Often produced from a number of different substances, including wheat, it's frequently used as a thickener. According to FALCPA, the food's label must state if it's made from wheat. Starch and dextrin can also be made from wheat. **Natural flavorings** can be the essence of any product derived from food products, and its function is for flavor, not nutrition (according to the Code of Federal Regulations, 21CFR101.22). Don't assume *natural flavoring* means "gluten free"; many contain gluten.

Guides to gluten-free grocery shopping can help you better navigate the aisles. *Gluten-Free Grocery Shopping Guide by Cecelia's Marketplace* written by Dr. Mara Matison and Mr. Dainis Matison and *Essential Gluten-Free Grocery Guide* by Triumph Dining are two guides that list ingredients gluten-free shoppers should avoid. (Triumph Dining also produces a guide to gluten-free dining.)

But don't be shy—pick up your phone and call a manufacturer from the store if you have a question the grocery clerk or the packaging can't clarify for you.

A great resource and an exhaustive list of ingredients often found in processed food labels is available at celiac.com/articles/182/1/Unsafe-Gluten-Free-Food-List-Unsafe-Ingredients/Page1.html.

Cross-Contamination

When you eat processed foods, you may run into difficulties because the food may be contaminated with gluten during the harvesting or manufacturing process. In fact, a recent study found that nearly a third of the 22 grains manufacturers labeled as gluten free actually were not. (This tested for gluten at or above 20 ppm.)

Also, manufacturers don't test their gluten-free grains for gluten. So you might purchase a gluten-free grain, like brown rice flour, at the grocery store, not realizing it was manufactured on equipment that also processed barley. Cross-contamination could have occurred during the milling.

When you're reading labels, check to see if the manufacturer mentions if the processing equipment was used to process gluten-containing ingredients. If it was, you probably should pass on that item.

> **FOOD FOR THOUGHT**
>
> Some companies, such as Whole Foods, bake their gluten-free goods in a separate facility from other baked goods to ensure gluten doesn't enter the processing plant.

Gluten Beyond Food

Unfortunately, gluten isn't limited to foods. Some medications contain glutenous fillers and may not list this information on the label. When it comes to prescriptions, talk to the pharmacist or be prepared to research the drug company's products.

You may need to consult your insurance company because drug choices will affect costs and coverage. Generics and brand-name products aren't made equally—one or the other could contain a gluten ingredient. If you're meeting with a doctor for tests, confirm that the doctor understands the importance of avoiding gluten before you accept any prescriptions.

Although some products are marketed as free of gluten, continue to read the labels. You can find products that suit your needs, but it might take a little detective work. If a label doesn't mention gluten, check the manufacturer's website or call to confirm the ingredients.

Packaged Gluten-Free Foods

Few gluten-free foods taste like the gluten-containing versions, but if gluten has been making you sick, that's probably the least of your worries right now. As you start your gluten-free journey, you might be surprised at the variety of prepackaged, gluten-free foods available to you.

The convenience of the gluten-free processed foods comes in handy as you transition. But keep in mind that as more manufacturers introduce gluten-free products, they're not necessarily leaving out the sugar, sodium, preservatives, and fillers. Gluten-free products may be healthier for you, but gluten-free processed foods are not as healthy as whole foods.

An occasional processed food treat is okay in moderation. But as you're reading the ingredient list, note how many items you recognize. If you read an ingredient and can't picture it in its natural state, you probably want to pass on that food.

Naturally Gluten-Free Foods

One of the easiest ways to avoid gluten is to purchase and cook foods in as close to their natural state as possible. Because they're minimally processed, naturally gluten-free foods often contain more nutrients for your body to enjoy.

So if you like hamburgers, for example, buy the ground meat and make your own patties. If you buy a premade hamburger, you run the risk that the manufacturer has added a filler, often a glutenous filler.

Following are a few categories of naturally gluten-free foods. Be sure to check the ingredients on the food you pick up, especially processed foods such as nuts or dairy, because manufacturers may add glutenous fillers.

- Beef

- Fish

- Pork—check processed lunchmeats

- Vegetables

- Fruits

- Dairy—check for malt additives

- Nuts—check for additional ingredients

- Beans

- Many herbs and spices—check for fillers in spice blends

- Condiments—check labels for indications of gluten

 FOOD FOR THOUGHT

Condiments that are generally gluten free include French's Mustard, Heinz Ketchup, most vinegars, Hellmann's Mayonnaise, Lea and Perrins Worcestershire Sauce, Miracle Whip, and Grey Poupon.

The Least You Need to Know

- Make lists and plan carefully, especially for your first trip to the grocery store after your diagnosis.

- If you have questions, ask at the store's customer service desk for help finding the location of gluten-free foods in the store or what the store's specific gluten-free labeling looks like.

- Don't know if the ingredients listed on the package are gluten free? Call the manufacturer. If you can't get a clear answer, don't buy the product.

- Shopping online can sometimes yield savings on gluten-free foods.

- Always read the labels, even with familiar foods. Manufacturers may change their ingredients without warning.

- Opt for fresh, whole foods—meats, vegetables, dairy—to naturally avoid gluten.

Quick and Easy Options

As you begin to shift to eating to gluten-free foods, you'll find that shopping for and preparing foods free of gluten takes a bit more planning. In this chapter, we help you get prepared and plan ahead, such as packing snacks. Shortcuts may be key at first, but soon you'll be well on your way to mastering the art of eating gluten free.

As you adjust to your new gluten-free lifestyle, explore flexible options to make your life easier. Discover a favorite and repeat. There's nothing wrong with figuring out what works for you and sticking to it. But do take time to explore ways to add variety, too.

In This Chapter

- More options for lunches
- Tips for advance preparation
- The importance of remaining flexible
- Adjusting to your gluten-free kitchen

A New Take on Sandwiches

Sandwiches—with their bread bookends—have been making you sick. And if you've looked into gluten-free breads, you know they can be more expensive than glutenous breads.

Fortunately, with a little planning and organization, eating gluten-free sandwiches doesn't have to be a big expense.

Gluten-Free Bread

If you like to eat bread, baking your own gluten-free bread is a great way to incorporate the taste you like and the freshness of homemade bread. With a little planning and experimentation, you can make your own gluten-free bread at home fairly easily.

Look for recipes that use rice flours, almond flour, or chickpea flour, or try some of the gluten-free bread mixes available. You might find that breads made with these flours look and taste somewhat different from wheat-based breads, but after a little getting used to, you'll find they offer a gluten-free solution to your sandwich problem.

If you want to make your own bread but are tight on time, consider purchasing a bread maker. This convenient appliance often comes with gluten-free recipes included. When purchasing a bread machine for gluten-free baking, consider ones that are programmable and allow for a cooling period. Also, review how easy it is to remove the paddle, and if the paddle will simply, but thoroughly, mix the ingredients.

Depending on how much bread you and your family eat, you may find making bread at home to be a welcome alternative to the high cost of store-bought bread. As you experiment, you may also come to really enjoy the bread-making process.

If baking at home isn't for you, yummy gluten-free breads are available, such as Udi's, Rudi's, and Schar brands. However, remember to always read the labels. These brands also make breads that contain gluten.

Beyond the Sandwich

Being gluten free opens all sorts of possibilities for delicious and nutritious lunches beyond the standard sandwich and frees you to think outside of the box. Because you have to change the *way* you've been eating, it's time to take a look at *what* you've been eating. One of the easiest ways to gluten-free eating is to choose recipes that normally don't have gluten.

Sure, you can buy the gluten-free breads, but consider these alternatives as well:

- Prepackaged gluten-free wraps made from safe grains

- Fresh lettuce wrapped around the sandwich goods (or reverse it by wrapping the meat or cheese around the green)

- Thinly sliced and grilled eggplant rolled up with meat and cheese

- Gluten-free tortillas, such as corn

- Gluten-free crepes with a savory filling

- Gluten-free pizza crust with your favorite toppings

- Gluten-free crackers topped with hummus or cheese

Some gluten-free wrap brands you might want to explore include La Tortilla Factory Millet and Teff Smart and Delicious Wraps or one of the Sandwich Petals variety. If you're not a fan of corn tortillas, try Udi's Plain Gluten-Free Tortillas or Rudi's Gluten-Free Tortillas.

GLUTEN GAFFE

Processed foods are processed foods. Don't overload on manufactured foods at the expense of your overall nutrition.

Be Prepared

Learning to eat gluten free might seem daunting at first, but preparation will become easier as you become more familiar with the foods you can eat and understand what you can't.

Don't complicate your life too much and make plans to cook and freeze dinner ahead for an entire month. But do take some time to figure out what meals or foods you can prepare ahead of time. An extra hour over the weekend focused on gluten-free food preparation can solve any potential last-minute food emergencies.

Cook Ahead

Pick a day of the week or weekend. Maybe it's only once a month or once every two weeks. But whenever you can, block out a few hours when you can cook several foods at once.

If you like burritos for lunch, spend an extra few minutes wrapping steamed corn tortillas around the filling, wrap the burritos with aluminum foil, date with a marker, and set in the freezer. On busy weekday mornings, grab a burrito from the freezer, and by lunchtime, the burrito—or whatever you've made ahead of time—will defrost by lunchtime.

Elizabeth sometimes makes extra of her weekend meals, such as her family's favorite gluten-free samosas, to freeze. These are easy to reheat for a tasty lunch or dinner treat during busy, on-the-go weeks. Try freezing food in individual portions for easier heating and serving. Individual servings also allow family members to pick and choose what they'd like to eat. Even if you forget to take the food out ahead of time, often the small-wrapped portions defrost quickly for dinner.

If you have a slow cooker, you can put it to work for you. Cook extra food, and even double recipes if you can. Then save half the food in the refrigerator or freezer for later in the week or month.

Maybe you cook your own spaghetti sauce on a stovetop. The next time you do, double the batch and freeze the second portion for future use.

If you have kids, get them involved in the preparation. Wrapping can be fun, and measuring ingredients can be educational. Having family involved in the cooking also helps underscore the importance of and allows for more discussion about gluten-free foods.

Fresh from the Freezer

In addition to providing an easy way to store the food you've prepared ahead of time, your freezer is also a great way to keep staples on hand.

When you're shopping, know what you and your family eat on a regular basis, purchase these foods in large quantities, and freeze part of what you buy. Lunchmeat is one item that freezes well. The night before you want to use it, transfer a portion from the freezer to the refrigerator to defrost.

Smoked salmon also freezes well and can be used for lunches and brunches. Defrost it in the refrigerator overnight.

Whether you buy or make your gluten-free bread, store it in the freezer. This keeps it fresh, and you can toast a slice at a time as needed. When you make homemade bread to freeze, it's best to slice it before you freeze it.

 TASTY TIDBIT

Toasting frozen bread changes the texture of it a bit, which might be helpful when you're adjusting to the slightly different texture gluten-free breads have.

You also can freeze homemade breads, muffins, scones, and other baked goods. These make quick and easy additions to lunches, but they can also become breakfasts and on-the-go snacks.

Or freeze just the dough of these baked goods, especially scones, and when you're craving something baked, you can thaw what you need, bake it, and enjoy. Pizza dough, for example, is great to have on hand in the freezer for lunches and dinners.

Cream cheese, goat's milk cheeses, and sheep's milk cheeses also freeze well. Cow's milk cheeses, however, do not freeze as well because the freezing process changes their protein structure. Cream cheese contains stabilizers that help it survive the freezing and thawing. Add a frozen bagel and some smoked salmon, and you've got lunch or brunch taken care of.

Homemade stocks and roasted vegetables are great to have in your freezer, too. They help you quickly and easily make lunch or dinner soups, or you can add them to casseroles. If you freeze roasted tomatoes, you can thaw them later for a divine tomato sauce.

Flexibility Is Key

We've all had those weeks when we're not able to get in the kitchen for a weekly food-preparation extravaganza, much less make dinner two nights in a row.

At least for a little while, your gluten-free life might not resemble your former life. That's okay. You've just found out the foods you've relied on—maybe for your entire life—have been making you sick. That may even include your all-time favorite foods. It's not going to be easy to adjust, but you will. Try to be flexible during your transition.

Think about the equipment you have in your kitchen now, and figure out how you can use it in support of your new diet. Make a healthy smoothie with your blender. Use your steamer to steam some broccoli to accompany a main dish. Chop and blend ingredients for a nutritional soup in your food processor. A toaster oven is great for broiling meat or melting open-faced cheese sandwiches.

If you have a recipe that calls for breadcrumbs, use gluten-free breadcrumbs. Are you supposed to thicken a gravy or stew with flour? Experiment with cornstarch, potato starch, or arrowroot flour. If a recipe calls for wheat for thickening, use half the amount in cornstarch, arrowroot flour, or potato starch, or use an equal amount of sweet rice flour.

After you've cleared out the gluten-free foods from your kitchen, get in there and start experimenting. The more you work in your kitchen, the more comfortable you'll be, and the more familiar you'll feel with preparing gluten-free foods.

It Pays to Stock Up

How flexible you are depends on how full your pantry is. To that end, we suggest you try to keep your pantry full of your go-to foods.

Maybe you've just discovered a pasta you and your family love. Next time you go shopping, buy a few extra boxes. You never know when you're going to have one of those nights when boiling water is the best you can do.

It's always a good idea to stock up on beans and rice. You can dress up these gluten-free fillers with cheeses, salsas, steamed greens, or just about anything else you can imagine. Add some leftover meat for extra protein.

If you frequent big-box retailers, start picking out where you can make the savings in the gluten-free foods you'll want to eat. For example, if you want to begin making more smoothies, maybe you can save money by buying large bags of frozen fruit.

In some big-box stores, you also can purchase grains, such as quinoa, in larger containers than at grocery stores and save money in the process.

To-Go Lunches and Snacks

Carrots, celery sticks, cucumbers, grapes, apple slices, and bananas are just a few snacks you easily can prep, pack, and take along for lunchtime meals or mid-afternoon snacks. Amie Valpone, editor-in-chief of The Healthy Apple (thehealthyapple.com), suggests bringing along hard-boiled eggs or avocados.

Elizabeth often buys Sabra snack-size containers of *hummus*. She pops a container into her purse with a handful of carrots whenever she knows she'll need a snack away from home. For a fantastic gluten-free hummus, check out our Healthy Hummus recipe in Chapter 15. Your snacks don't need to be elaborate, just filling.

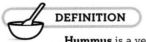

> **DEFINITION**
>
> **Hummus** is a vegetable dip made from sesame-seed paste, chickpeas, garlic, and lemon juice. It can also be used as a spread.

Think about the snack foods you ate before going gluten free. You may have enjoyed crackers, pretzels, roasted nuts, and cereals. The glutenous versions of these foods may not be an option any more, but lots of great gluten-free alternatives are available.

Try these quick snacks:

- Glutino crackers (glutino.com) or Blue Diamond Nut Thins or Nut Chips (bluediamond.com/index.cfm?navid=21)

- Allergen-free snacks from Enjoy Life (enjoylifefoods.com)

- Gluten-free pretzels, such as Glutino or Ener-G (ener-g.com)

- Snack bars, such as LÄRABARs (larabar.com) or KIND bars (kindsnacks.com)

- Rice Chex (chex.com/Recipes/GlutenFree.aspx) or other gluten-free cereals, such as those from Nature's Path (naturespath.com)

- Homemade snacks (check out Chapter 18 for recipes, including Gluten-Free Crackers and Chickpea Flatbread)

- Plain fruits and vegetables, including grapes and celery sticks

- Nuts and seeds—a handful of one kind of nuts or seeds, or mix up your snack with a variety

- Snack-size cheese bites

- Popcorn (if there's a flavor added, check the ingredients list to avoid gluten)

If you have access to boiling water or a microwave at work or school, experiment with prepackaged noodles or rice bowls. Gluten-free options are available at grocery and health food stores. Some examples include the following:

- Annie Chun's products (anniechun.com), such as Rice Express Sprouted Brown Sticky Rice microwavable bowls

- Amy's products (amys.com/products/product-categories/gluten-free), including the Bean and Rice Burritos, often available in the frozen foods section, and canned soups

- Tasty Bite (tastybite.com), for heat-and-eat gluten-free Indian food options

Gluten-free baked goods are another great portable snack. Protein-packed muffins made with almond flour, nuts, and seeds are easy to bake, package, transport, and eat. Jeanette's Lemon Poppy Seed Scones in Chapter 18 are also convenient and can be customized with different flavors.

Baked goods often freeze well, too. Make a double or triple batch and freeze the extras so you have a snack to bring along.

Breakfast for Dinner

Being flexible also might mean adjusting your ideas about which foods to eat for breakfast, lunch, and dinner. Why not enjoy an omelet with mushrooms, cheese, and sautéed greens for dinner? If you have kids, creating a weekly "breakfast for dinner" night can be a fun way to involve them in meal planning.

Got extra gluten-free bread? Try mixing up a savory version of French toast. Like crepes? You can dress up gluten-free crepes or buckwheat pancakes for dinner with steamed vegetables and melted cheeses. Consider making Chapter 13's Cornmeal Pancakes as a side for eggs. Or fix polenta with soft-boiled eggs.

Dinner isn't the only meal you can switch up. Try sweet potatoes for breakfast with a smidgen of brown sugar and butter for an early morning pick-me-up.

 TASTY TIDBIT

> Switch out a flavoring when you can to add variety. If you're browning beef for several meals, for example, don't add any seasonings until you heat the meat for the meal at hand.

The point is to mix and match what you can, when you can. You're learning what you can and can't eat, so it's okay to repeat meals a few times in one week, especially when you find something gluten free you like. Be flexible and have fun with your meals. Gluten-free eating may be hard at first, but we have no doubt you'll manage.

A New Way to Cook

One of the hardest parts of going gluten free is giving up those favorite recipes that have been in your family for generations. Or maybe you love the way a certain restaurant makes French toast. Or there's that guilty pleasure you have, a childhood treat that provides comfort when you're seriously stressed out.

If you've just been diagnosed, sometimes the cravings for the foods you're familiar with are just plain hard.

Now that you're gluten free, you might wonder if it's possible to re-create some of your favorite foods in your own kitchen. If you're not an experienced cook, the prospect might seem daunting. Even if you're comfortable in the kitchen, you might be worried about using unfamiliar ingredients.

Gluten-free cooking can be challenging, but it doesn't have to be. Approach it with a spirit of exploration and discovery, and you may find meals you like just as much as—or more than!—your old favorites.

Appealing to the Senses

The sense of taste is one of the greatest human pleasures. Eating wouldn't be such a fabulous proposition if we couldn't tell the difference between sauerkraut and chocolate-chip cookies. You may be wondering if you'll still be able to enjoy your sense of taste now that you must eat gluten free. After all, hasn't everyone said that gluten-free foods have no flavor?

Remember that our senses of taste and smell are linked and that smell is associated with memory. Your favorite chicken pot pie might taste good not just because of the flavors on your tongue, but also because of the savory aromas you inhale and the memories those smells trigger. It's no wonder we're not thrilled when faced with the task of changing our eating habits. We may be dispensing with our memory.

You might not be able to replicate the exact taste and texture of your favorite foods, but what if you could create some of the smells that bring back good memories? What if you take the building blocks of some of your recipes, remove the offending gluten, and still retain some of the smell that connects to your memories?

Here are some suggestions as you start thinking about how to recreate your favorite foods. These suggestions are also important to keep in mind when you crave a gluten-filled favorite food.

- Chew your food more, which helps you release more of its flavor.

- Utilize your favorite herbs and spices—maybe cumin or cinnamon—to add a familiar zing to simple meals.

- Start with naturally flavorful, unprocessed foods.

- Experiment with gluten-free brines or marinades that add a distinct and flavorful pop to foods.

FOOD FOR THOUGHT

The world is home to more than 10,000 unique smells, and on average, each tongue contains 5,000 taste buds. That's more than enough to keep your nose and taste buds busy with tasty gluten-free foods.

Get Ready to Experiment

You might be ready to cook up a storm right now, but take a look at some of your former favorite foods first. Are they simple to re-create? If it's as easy as substituting rice flour lasagna noodles for semolina lasagna noodles, you may be able to adjust the recipe easily with good results. But if you're new to gluten-free baking, keep in mind that you could need time to experiment with the different flours before you're able to get the tastes and textures you're looking for.

Determine if you can try to substitute an ingredient here or there. Maybe you can swap out breadcrumbs for crumbled gluten-free potato chips. Will the gluten-free Bisquick perform like the glutenous Bisquick? Try it and see.

It might be that you need to dispense with trying to make your grandmother's famous side dish that included a topping of crumbled Ritz crackers. You may never be able to re-create what grandmother's tasted like, but that's okay. Make it your own instead. Add your own twist to the recipe so generations from now will never know it contained gluten to begin with.

Be prepared for failures. Often recipes for gluten-free breads include sweeter ingredients to mask the grainier tasting flours. Those may not be for you. Other flours have such a different consistency that you might never truly replicate the texture of the sandwich bread you hope for.

When it comes to gluten-free baking, experiment to find what recipes appeal to you. In Chapter 18, we give you a recipe for All-Purpose Gluten-Free Flour Blend, should you want to replace your recipes with a one-to-one flour substitute.

Several gluten-free flour blends are available, too. When you're just starting out, buy a few flour blend mixes to try. If you have time, test a recipe out twice, with two different flour blends so you can compare the tastes to determine what you like best.

Feeling Comfortable in the Kitchen

Not sure how to tell your measuring spoon from your measuring cup? Never had to tie any apron strings? We've all been there. Maybe no one taught you to cook, or maybe you were only taught to defrost or to press start on the microwave.

The instructions for the recipes in this book are just a bit longer than the directions you've seen on packaged foods. Most of the recipes are pretty easy to follow; some, like the French buttercream frosting, are a bit more difficult at first, but the taste is so divine it's worth the extra effort.

If you're a novice cook, we recommend doing a search on YouTube or Google to find video instructions for basic cooking and kitchen skills. Lots of culinary instruction videos are available for free online. You might also want to consider taking a cooking class to help you master basic skills.

Keep in mind that learning to cook takes time, and it's best to start with small, manageable tasks. Hosting a dinner party for 12 is not the best time to attempt new recipes or techniques. Also, you might want to avoid any celebratory parties until you've mastered baking a gluten-free cake. You can always serve ice cream and other, naturally gluten-free desserts.

 TASTY TIDBIT

> When starting out, focus on simple meals—for example, broiled chicken, steamed green beans, and rice—then start adding some pizzazz. Experiment with marinades, brines, spices, and herbs until you find a flavor combination that leaves your old menus in the dust. Add a squeeze of lemon to your cooking for an unexpected zing.

Learning to cook with new ingredients will take practice. Try recipes more than once, and learn from your mistakes. Elizabeth once baked a cake for her husband's birthday that sank in the middle. Frosting pooled in the indentation and didn't harden. Fortunately, it was a family dinner with children who were more interested in eating cake than how it might look.

She practiced the cake a couple more times before unveiling it at the extended family's Easter meal. The result? She left that meal promising the recipe to most of the folks at the table, none of whom could believe the cake was gluten free.

Even if you know how to cook, some gluten-free ingredients might be unfamiliar to you or hard to find. But you also might be surprised at how much you *can* cook that's gluten free and doesn't require additional, hard-to-find ingredients. If you do discover a substitution you like for a recipe, make a note of it and repeat it whenever you can.

Tweaking recipes is a standard practice for most home cooks. Don't be afraid to add your own flair; you don't have to follow a recipe exactly for a dish to taste amazing. The only caveat is to follow measurements for baking exactly. Cooking is art, but baking is more science—especially when it comes to gluten-free goods.

Here are some hints to make your culinary journey more successful:

- Always read the recipe through to the end.
- Double check that you have all the ingredients.
- Don't have all the ingredients? Figure out suitable substitutes.
- Make a note—in the cookbook—of any substitutes or recipe changes.
- Tweak and keep tweaking until you've found the flavor you want.

Pick a weekend or day when you aren't pressed for time to practice new recipes. If you like, invite a few close friends or family members to sample your creations.

The Least You Need to Know

- Look for nutritious alternatives to breads when making sandwiches. Lettuce or gluten-free wraps are a good place to start.
- A well-stocked refrigerator and freezer can help you transition to gluten-free eating more easily.
- Flexibility in meals and menu planning helps you adjust to your new gluten-free diet.
- Be prepared to experiment. Learning to cook gluten-free is a process of trial and error. Try to make it a fun process.

CHAPTER 8

Gluten-Free Menu Planning

When you're suffering from a serious health issue, such as gluten intolerance, you need to take action immediately. The more gluten you eat, the more your villus suffers. It's imperative for you to get organized and figure out what to eat for the next couple weeks. We've made it easy, with the recipes in Part 4. We also included a 2-week meal plan in this chapter to help you get started.

By the time you're ready to explore other gluten-free cookbooks, you'll have a better sense of what kind of foods you like and want to incorporate into your gluten-free diet.

In This Chapter

- Tips for getting—and staying—organized
- Choosing the right recipes for you
- Creating a gluten-free menu
- Two weeks of gluten-free meals

Getting Organized

Prior to your diagnosis, you might have handled meal planning and eating in many different ways. Maybe you're the type of person who has a shelf full of meticulously organized cookbooks with notes in the margins. Perhaps you're already accustomed to planning ahead, shopping with a list, and sticking to a plan. If so, the transition to eating gluten-free may come easily to you.

However, if you're more prone to playing it by ear and eating on the go, you'll need to adjust your habits. Eating gluten-free takes some forethought, especially at first. Even if it feels regimented and difficult, force yourself to think through what your meals will be for the coming weeks. Write them down. Make a list of ingredients to buy. Be sure you set aside time to cook.

Once you develop a routine, you can introduce more flexibility. For now, though, it's important to be organized for your health.

Moving Gluten Out of Focus

If gluten has had a starring role in your life, it's time to demote it. Just like you cleared out glutenous foods from your pantry and kitchen, you also need to remove cookbooks that may emphasize wheat and its cousins.

It wasn't long into gluten-free eating that Elizabeth realized organization would help her stay focused on her new diet. She moved her old go-to cookbooks so they were no longer the first things she reached for. Gluten-free cookbooks and a three-ring binder with recipes clipped from gluten-free magazines took their place. With the temptation of gluten cooking out of reach, gluten-free recipes were more in the spotlight.

You probably have your own methods of selecting and storing recipes. Whatever it is, set those old, glutenous recipes aside and replace them with gluten-free recipes and cooking ideas that interest you.

If you don't have any organizational methods in place, take time to set up something. Maybe select a nice binder with dividers, or use file folders to collect recipes and notes on gluten-free eating. This is a lifestyle shift, so embrace it and treat it in a way that honors your commitment to you and your health.

 FOOD FOR THOUGHT

Gluten free is a growing trend. Nearly 30 percent of adults are interested in cutting out gluten from their diet. Gluten free has blossomed into a $4.2 billion industry, with diners placing more than 200 million gluten-free restaurant orders between January and September 2012, according to a January 2013 survey by NPD Group.

As you go through your existing cookbooks and recipes, sort them into two piles—keep or give away.

Keep …

- Magazines with allergen-free recipes.

- Cookbooks that have a wide range of recipes so gluten isn't in every recipe.

- Different cuisine cookbooks to spice up your diet.

Donate or give away …

- Cookbooks that focus on bread or bread making.

- Cookbooks about grains.

- Pasta cookbooks because even if you eat gluten-free pasta, now is a good time to beef up your nutrition.

Great Gluten-Free Resources

The internet is a fantastic source of gluten-free recipes, tips, and advice. Elana's Pantry (elanaspantry.com) has become Elizabeth's go-to favorite. Many of the recipes on Elana's site call for only a handful of ingredients and are simple, nutritious, and delicious.

By following Elana's blog and other gluten-free websites, Elizabeth was able to discover new favorites for her and her family. She quickly learned about rice pancakes; substituting applesauce for eggs; almond flour crust; and agar flakes, which are vegan and great for thickening.

TASTY TIDBIT

For more gluten-free bloggers, check out celiaccentral.org/Resources/Gluten-Free-Bloggers/125.

You may find gluten-free bloggers a valuable resource for recipes and food ideas, too. Here are a few recommended by the National Foundation for Celiac Awareness (NFCA):

- Be Free for Me (befreeforme.com/blog) offers product reviews and some recipes.

- Best Life Gluten Free (bestlifeglutenfree.com) provides lots of recipes.

- College Student with Celiac (collegestudentwithceliac.wordpress.com) is written for college students by a college student.

- Celiac Central: Bits and Bites (celiaccentral.wordpress.com) is the blog written by the staff of the NFCA.

Making and sharing recipes from food blogs could even inspire someone else. Elizabeth once brought a dessert to a party hosted by a woman who was inching her way into gluten-free eating. A taste of Elizabeth's dessert convinced the hostess that gluten free would be okay. Elizabeth passed along the recipe, and the next time she was at her friend's house, her friend had tried several other recipes from the same food blog and was well on her way to full-time gluten freedom.

Make a List

We know, sometimes making lists can feel like a chore. But really, a shopping list helps you get organized when it comes to gluten-free eating. Some people create their own templates they copy and print for each week. Other people have a clipboard for each grocery store. A variety of smartphone apps are available for making lists, too. Whatever you like and works for you, use it.

Why are lists so important? Because in gluten-free eating, you'll rarely find one store that fits all your needs. Maybe the sweet rice flour comes from store A, while the gluten-free pizza crusts are only available at store B. Store C is the one you'll shop at for buying bulk items or stocking up on pasta.

Elizabeth carries a master list divided by store with the items she needs to buy written under each store name. She notes specific brands on this list as well. Instead of "pasta," she lists "Bionaturae gluten-free pasta."

Elizabeth may buy all her vegetables and fruits from a grocery store and stock up on baking items from the cooperative food store. However, if she finds the flour she wants at the grocery store, she can cross that off her master list and skip the coop stop.

This "master list" method might work for you, or you could make a separate list for each store. Figure out whatever works for you and stick with it. It'll save you a lot of hassles.

 FOOD FOR THOUGHT

Lists are also handy at tax time. Staple receipts to your grocery list, and talk to the tax man. If you're diagnosed as having celiac disease, you may receive tax deductions for expenses for gluten-free foods and supplies. Check out the IRS website (irs.gov/taxtopics/tc502.html) for more details, and consult a tax specialist or accountant.

Things happen, and life is busy enough that taking a few minutes to write down a few items can save you loads of time in the long run—especially if you have to run around town to buy everything you need.

Choosing Recipes

One of the reasons we've included more than 70 recipes in this book is to help you begin choosing and planning gluten-free meals. We encourage you to experiment with these and other recipes and determine what nutrients you need to emphasize in your diet.

What Can't You Eat?

As you probably know all too well, if you have gluten intolerance, you may have to avoid certain other foods, too. Starting there can help you determine what you can eat. If you're cooking for others, you'll want to take their dietary restrictions into consideration as well.

Elizabeth can eat nuts, but not peanuts. She discovered almond flour and loves the taste of almond flour in crusts. But she has extended family members who can't eat any nuts, so she adjusts the recipes accordingly or doesn't use almond flour when they are around. Instead of a quiche with an almond flour crust, for example, she'll make gluten-free crepes with a similar vegetable filling.

What Do You Need to Eat?

As a gluten-intolerant eater, you may have experienced malabsorption of nutrients. In fact, you may have been told you need to regain some of the vitamins or minerals your body has been missing or not processing well.

The U.S. government requires grains to be enriched with vitamins and minerals, but as a person suffering from gluten intolerance, you may not have been able to process those vitamins and minerals to benefit your body. You might need to increase your intake of foods that provide the vitamin B range—B_1, B_2, B_3, B_9, and B_{12}—and vitamin D.

Chapter 2 provides specifics regarding nutrition, but remember to try to plan balanced meals made from whole food ingredients.

Planning Your Gluten-Free Menu

Habits are hard to break, especially when it comes to your stomach. Approach your new way of eating with a positive attitude, and keep in mind that eating gluten free helps your body be at its best.

Take Time

Committing to a dietary change for 2 weeks can help you reset your eating habits. We suggest a 2-week period during which you don't anticipate any obvious stressors—no upcoming weddings to plan, no big vacations on the calendar, no big tests to take.

Plan to spend time looking at new recipes to determine how best to fit these new foods into your week. Then, spend some time at the grocery store shopping for your ingredients. The more time you can take at the beginning, the easier it will be for you as the week gets busier.

 TASTY TIDBIT

We've all been there. You have the best intentions to run home and cook dinner, but a meeting runs late, so you think about grabbing something on the way home. However, if you've planned ahead, you'll have plenty of nutritious, gluten-free food in the refrigerator, freezer, or pantry you can eat instead.

Before You Begin …

You don't have to fit all the recipes in Part 4 into a 2-week menu plan. We've done it for you—with a few added suggestions—so you can see everything you can eat on a gluten-free diet. Maybe it's easier for you to try just two or three new recipes a week. Perhaps you can substitute past dinner or breakfast favorites with new gluten-free substitutions and then just gradually integrate these new recipes.

We know it can be daunting for you—for anyone!—to try a new menu plan. So if you decide to take bits and pieces and load up the rest of the time on plain fruits, veggies, and meats—the things that are obviously and have always been gluten free—that's fine. Find a few favorite, non-gluten fruits, vegetables, and meats, and be sure you always have at least two or three quick meals you can put together or warm up when you most need them. Then, as you become more comfortable in your lifestyle, add new recipes, try new dishes, and experiment.

That's worked for Jeanette. As long as she focuses on vegetables and fruits and ensure her pantry is always stocked, she easily can throw together a salad, toss a stir-fry, or fix a quick fruit salad.

A Two-Week Gluten-Free Menu Plan

Many of the selections in this menu plan come from the recipes in this book. We've also added some general foods you can prepare without a recipe to add some flavor and ease to your plan.

Use this 2-week menu plan as a starting point, and change it depending on the season, upcoming holidays, or busy weeks. Use the weekends to make more time-intensive dishes, such as Banana

Bread (Chapter 18), Cornmeal Pancakes (Chapter 13), or Mama's Meatloaf (Chapter 16), and double the recipe. Put half aside, and freeze what you can to build a cushion for busier weeks.

> **TASTY TIDBIT**
>
> Besides shopping for food items, be sure to include different sizes of freezer bags, aluminum foil, and storage containers. When you make a double batch of a recipe, you'll be able to freeze the extra portions easily.

Week 1

Start out simple and start adding to the complexity of your menu. Following are some ideas of how to plan your first week of gluten-free eating. You'll need to make time to plan, shop for, and cook these dishes, so factor that in. Between meals, add fresh fruits, vegetables, or nuts for nutritious snacking or additional sides for meals. If you have other dietary restrictions, please consult a nutritionist, and feel free to adjust for your needs and any allergies.

Now, get cooking!

Day 1:

- **Breakfast:** gluten-free oatmeal with seasonal fruit and honey
- **Snack:** 1 cup mixed nuts
- **Lunch:** Crunchy Asian Quinoa Salad (Chapter 14)
- **Snack:** 1 handful carrots with Ranch Dressing (Chapter 14)
- **Dinner:** Crab Cakes (Chapter 16) with a mixed-greens side salad with Honey Mustard Dressing (Chapter 14) and 1 cup fresh fruit

Day 2:

- **Breakfast:** Cornmeal Pancakes (Chapter 13)
- **Snack:** 1 cup mixed nuts
- **Lunch:** gluten-free turkey lunchmeat, alfalfa sprouts, and avocado wrapped in a corn tortilla with Basic Mayonnaise (Chapter 15) and 1 cup fresh fruit
- **Snack:** 1 serving applesauce
- **Dinner:** Mama's Meatloaf (Chapter 16) with a mixed-greens side salad with Ranch Dressing (Chapter 14) and 1 baked sweet potato

Day 3:

- **Breakfast:** Cinnamon Maple Quinoa Cereal (Chapter 13)

- **Snack:** 1 cup mixed nuts

- **Lunch:** open-faced melted cheese and gluten-free turkey lunchmeat on gluten-free bread with a side of Roasted Asparagus Salad (Chapter 14) and 1 piece of fruit

- **Snack:** sliced cucumber with Healthy Hummus (Chapter 15)

- **Dinner:** broiled salmon fillet with a side of asparagus salad with sautéed spinach and Rice Pilaf (Chapter 16)

Day 4:

- **Breakfast:** hot buckwheat cereal or cream of rice

- **Snack:** 1 cup fresh fruit

- **Lunch:** Basic Risotto (Chapter 16) with steamed vegetables with 1 piece fresh fruit

- **Snack:** 1 cup mixed nuts

- **Dinner:** Arroz con Pollo (Chapter 16) with a mixed-greens side salad and Balsamic Vinaigrette (Chapter 14) with 1 cup mixed fruit

Day 5:

- **Breakfast:** Sausage, Cheese, and Spinach Breakfast Casserole (Chapter 13) with 1 piece fresh fruit

- **Snack:** Grain-Free Peanut Butter Granola (Chapter 13) with 1 cup yogurt

- **Lunch:** Healthy Hummus (Chapter 15) with Gluten-Free Crackers (Chapter 18) with slices of carrots, celery, and cucumber

- **Snack:** 1 cup mixed nuts

- **Dinner:** Leftovers of any main meal from earlier in the week with a mixed-greens side salad and 1 cup fresh fruit

Day 6:

- **Breakfast:** Banana Bread (Chapter 18) with a fruit smoothie

- **Snack:** 1 gluten-free bagel with cream cheese

- **Lunch:** gluten-free turkey lunchmeat, mixed greens, and red pepper slices in a corn tortilla and 1 piece fresh fruit

- **Snack:** carrots with Healthy Hummus (Chapter 15)

- **Dinner:** Basic Pizza Crust (Chapter 18) with your choice of gluten-free toppings and vegetables

Day 7:

- **Breakfast:** Zucchini Chocolate Bread (Chapter 18) with 1 cup fresh fruit; make a batch of Basic Gluten-Free Pasta Noodle dough (Chapter 17) for use later in the week

- **Snack:** Grain-Free Peanut Butter Granola (Chapter 13) with 1 cup yogurt

- **Lunch:** Basic Risotto (Chapter 16) with vegetables or a mixed-greens side salad

- **Snack:** 1 cup mixed nuts

- **Dinner:** Salmon *en Papillote* (Chapter 16) with Simple Kale Salad (Chapter 14) and 1 piece fresh fruit

DEFINITION

En Papillote is a French term that refers to wrapping food inside oiled parchment paper. As the food—fish or meat—steams inside the paper, the parchment paper expands and balloons or puffs out. When serving, slit open the paper to reveal the cooked food.

Week 2

You've been eating gluten-free for a week! Did you even notice the missing gluten? Now let's add a few other recipes and make plans for leftovers.

Day 1:

- **Breakfast:** gluten-free oatmeal with raisins and fruit

- **Snack:** Grain-Free Peanut Butter Granola (Chapter 13) with 1 cup yogurt

- **Lunch:** Caesar Salad with Homemade Croutons (Chapter 14) with grilled chicken breast

- **Snack:** carrots with 1 cup Healthy Hummus (Chapter 15)

- **Dinner:** Braised Short Ribs (Chapter 16) with Cornbread (Chapter 18) and Steamed Broccoli and 1 piece fresh fruit

Day 2:

- **Breakfast:** Buckwheat Buttermilk Pancakes with Strawberry Balsamic Syrup (Chapter 13)
- **Snack:** 1 cup yogurt sprinkled with mixed nuts
- **Lunch:** Leftovers of Braised Short Ribs and Cornbread
- **Snack:** 1 cup fresh fruit
- **Dinner:** Curried Sweet Potato Soup (Chapter 16) with Gluten-Free Crackers (Chapter 18) and a mixed-greens side salad and your choice salad dressing from Chapter 14; make extra soup for freezing

Day 3:

- **Breakfast:** Gluten-Free Crepes with Caramelized Bananas (Chapter 13) sprinkled with your favorite nuts
- **Snack:** 1 cup mixed nuts
- **Lunch:** Gluten-Free Crackers (Chapter 18) with Walnut Tofu Pate and Spread (Chapter 15) and a mixed-greens side salad and Asian Ginger Dressing (Chapter 14) and 1 cup fresh fruit
- **Snack:** Grain-Free Peanut Butter Granola (Chapter 13) with 1 cup yogurt
- **Dinner:** grilled fish with Crunchy Asian Quinoa Salad (Chapter 14)

Day 4:

- **Breakfast:** gluten-free oatmeal with raisins, seasonal fruit, and maple syrup
- **Snack:** 1 cup yogurt mixed with fresh fruit
- **Lunch:** gluten-free lunchmeat, avocado, and cucumber slices in a gluten-free wrap with 1 piece fresh fruit
- **Snack:** 1 cup mixed nuts
- **Dinner:** Cheese Ravioli (Chapter 17) with a Simple Kale Salad (Chapter 14) and 1 cup fresh fruit

Day 5:

- **Breakfast:** Grain-Free Peanut Butter Granola (Chapter 13) with milk (or a milk substitute) and 1 cup fresh berries

- **Snack:** 1 cup yogurt mixed with fresh fruit

- **Lunch:** gluten-free lunchmeat, Basic Mayonnaise (Chapter 15), and lettuce on toasted gluten-free bread and Kale Chips (Chapter 15) with fresh fruit

- **Snack:** 1 cup Healthy Hummus (Chapter 15) with cut carrots, celery, or your favorite vegetables

- **Dinner:** Chicken, Cauliflower, and Potato Curry (Chapter 16) with steamed rice and fresh fruit salad

Day 6:

- **Breakfast:** Cranberry Orange Muffins (Chapter 18) and a side cup of yogurt and fresh fruit; make extra muffins and freeze them for next week

- **Snack:** 1 cup mixed nuts

- **Lunch:** Curried Sweet Potato Soup (Chapter 16) and sliced cucumbers and 1 piece fruit

- **Snack:** Grain-Free Peanut Butter Granola (Chapter 13) with 1 cup yogurt

- **Dinner:** Stuffed Peppers (Chapter 16) and Rice Pilaf (Chapter 16) and a mixed-greens side salad

Day 7:

- **Breakfast:** Lemon Poppy Seed Scones (Chapter 18) with yogurt and fresh fruit

- **Lunch:** Meat Pierogis (Chapter 17) and Roasted Asparagus Salad (Chapter 14) with 1 piece fresh fruit; make additional pierogis for freezing for lunches next week

- **Dinner:** Spaghetti Marinara with Homemade Meatballs (Chapter 17) served with a mixed-greens side salad and Balsamic Vinaigrette (Chapter 14) and mixed fruit salad

Week 3 and Moving Forward

Take what you've planned and cooked after 2 weeks, and assess what you need to change, add, or delete. Build on the process you started 2 weeks previously and make more lists, double more recipes, and freeze more standby foods. Embrace that you're well on your way to gluten-free eating for life!

The Least You Need to Know

- Get rid of old cookbooks that celebrate wheat and its glutenous cousins. Keep cookbooks or recipes that use whole foods.
- Make or purchase a special notebook to keep gluten-free recipes and other notes about your new diet. Place it prominently in your kitchen.
- Lists, lists, lists will help you sort through all the different foods you may need to purchase. Don't get frustrated—get organized!
- Familiar tastes—and re-creating those tastes—are important as you move into gluten-free eating.
- Use our menu plan or create your own to get yourself in the good habit of planning ahead and resetting your eating habits.

Living a Gluten-Free Life

In Part 3, we take you out of your kitchen and on the road as you survive and thrive in your new gluten-free life.

We help you find gluten-free items on restaurant menus and ensure you have something safe to eat while eating at the homes of friends and family. We even offer advice on gluten-free eating while traveling. We suggest safe ways to host a party and entertain your friends—and introduce them to some of your newfound favorite gluten-free dishes.

If you have children who need to avoid gluten, we address that, too, with insight on dealing with schools and teachers, as well as school celebrations.

In the final chapter of Part 3, we suggest ways for thriving while eating gluten free. We've been there, and we have plenty of ideas on how to beat your cravings for your old favorite glutenous foods.

CHAPTER 9

Gluten Free Away from Home

After Elizabeth started eating a gluten-free diet, she realized she was shying away from dining out at restaurants, avoiding parties, and making excuses for not traveling. You might have similar feelings and even fear eating outside the safety of your gluten-free kitchen.

But you needn't worry. By taking a few precautions when you eat out, you can enjoy being social again. In this chapter, we look at how you can be successfully gluten free away from home and give you pointers on how to approach the restaurant menu, your server, and even the chef if necessary. We also take a look at eating while visiting the homes of friends and family. And so you can ensure you avoid gluten while farther away from home, we give you some tips for being gluten free on the road.

In This Chapter

- Eating out gluten free
- Dining with friends
- Gluten free on the road
- Accidental gluten encounters

Gluten Free in Restaurants

Dining out when you're gluten intolerant can be a scary thought. You might even feel like you're heading into a minefield filled with gluten-laden explosives.

Eating every single meal for the rest of your life in the safety of your kitchen isn't realistic, so you need to know how to eat out and avoid gluten.

The good news is that many restaurants these days list gluten-free items on their menus. But you still might encounter places where gluten is all over the menu, and your server might not even know what gluten is. We can help.

Do Your Research

One of the most important things you can do to avoid gluten when dining out is to spend some time checking out the restaurant and its menu. You may even want to call or visit the restaurant before you actually eat there. Amie Valpone, editor-in-chief of The Healthy Apple, recommends you "always call ahead before you go to the restaurant and then be sure to ask your waiter to speak with the chef so there is no cross-contamination." She often speaks directly to the chef to ensure her gluten-free needs are understood.

Start by researching a restaurant and determining what you think you can eat from the menu before you go to meet with the chef. Review the menu online so you can ask specific questions and show you're taking your intolerance seriously. Many local restaurants and chains now indicate on menus what dishes and sauces are naturally gluten-free and which can be altered to be gluten-free. Fleming's Steakhouse, Carrabba's Italian Grill, and Olive Garden Italian Restaurant do a nice job of this.

Schedule time a couple days before you plan to eat at the restaurant to visit and meet with the manager and chef. Plan your visit so you're not there during the busy breakfast, lunch, or dinner rushes. Keep the conversation polite, but also bring information about gluten intolerance and be prepared to leave the information. If the chef and staff are agreeable and willing to take your gluten requests seriously, make a reservation so they can note in your reservation your food intolerances and any specific requests.

FOOD FOR THOUGHT

The Gluten Intolerance Group (GIG) and the National Foundation for Celiac Awareness (NFCA) provide information to educate others, including restaurants, about gluten. Visit gluten.net/Programs/industry-programs/gluten-free-food-service or CeliacCentral.org to learn more.

If you can't visit beforehand, review the menu online. Calling the restaurant and talking to the manager or chef over the phone is another option if you can't go there in person.

Gratitude is a key component, whether you speak to the chef in person or on the phone. Spend time letting the restaurant staff know you appreciate their attention and accommodation of your dietary restriction. If you can, send a letter to the restaurant's owner or the corporate office afterward to let them know how much you appreciated the restaurant staff making an effort to accommodate your intolerance. Be sure to give your waitstaff a nice tip, too.

Always be polite. It's easy to get frustrated when restaurant staff don't understand your food limitations. Even though celiac disease and gluten intolerance is increasingly in the news, many people still don't understand it. Be polite but firm in explaining what you can and can't eat.

Speak Up

If you haven't had a chance to speak with the chef before you visit a restaurant, all is not lost. When you arrive, don't be shy about making your gluten-free needs known. Talk with your host or hostess as you're being seated. Mention that you can't have foods with gluten and that cross-contamination is also a problem for you. Ask if he or she knows how chefs handle food allergies and special requests. If not, your next resource is your server.

When you meet your server, tell them you're gluten intolerant so it puts them on alert. Ask if the restaurant has a special gluten-free menu or if the regular menu lists gluten-free items.

> **FOOD FOR THOUGHT**
>
> In its 2013 industry forecast, the National Restaurant Association cites gluten-free menu items as one of its top trends of the year, including nonwheat noodles and pastas, quinoa, and buckwheat.

If your server knows the menu and ingredients the chef uses, he or she might be able to recommend some gluten-free options for you. Or they might point out some items on the menu the kitchen can make without glutenous ingredients. Otherwise, he or she might go back to the kitchen and ask the manager or chef.

If the manager or chef comes out of the kitchen to speak with you, be polite, gracious, and complimentary. Explain that you have difficulty with gluten and would like to know how a certain dish is prepared. Also ask if the knives or other utensils could be washed before your dish is prepared to prevent cross-contamination. It might take some time to explain, but you'll feel more secure that you've approached the right people.

Short of preparing your meal yourself in your gluten-free kitchen, you'll never be 100 percent sure your meal is made as you'd prepare it. And unfortunately, the information about your gluten-free request might not stick. For example, Elizabeth and her husband have a favorite place they like to eat. They've had the same gluten conversation with the owners of the restaurant, who sometimes also prepare the food. "No bread" is written across order after order, but when others besides the owners prepare the food, salads sometimes arrive with croutons sprinkled throughout, and sandwiches arrive with bread.

Confusion happens sometimes. Being clear while also being polite and friendly makes the experience better for you and helps others learn a little more about gluten intolerance.

If you've made your request clear, you certainly can send back any glutenous food you receive and ask for a replacement dish without the offending ingredient. Be sure to explain—nicely—that simply removing the croutons from your salad, for example, won't work because even the smallest cross-contamination could make you ill.

And don't just assume something on the menu is gluten-free. Jeanette recently ordered spicy tuna rolls at a sushi restaurant, thinking they'd be safe. She took one bite and discovered panko bread-crumbs in the rolls. And this is after she asked for gluten-free tamari sauce.

Gluten-Free Fast Food?

Yes, you can find gluten-free fast food. But don't always count on it. As with non-fast-food restaurants, it's a good idea to do some research ahead of time on the fast-food places you think might have gluten-free options you can eat.

The first place to start your investigation is online. If you haven't looked at restaurant websites lately, you might be surprised to find pages of allergy information provided. Bookmark the appropriate pages, and make notes on which foods you can eat at which restaurants. If you want, print the information and keep it in your car. If you have a smartphone, you can look up the restaurant information when you're out and about and deciding where to eat.

One great resource in the restaurant search is the Gluten Intolerance Group, which offers a list of restaurants that voluntarily participate in the GIG's Gluten-Free Restaurant Awareness Program. Learn more at glutenfreerestaurants.org.

 TASTY TIDBIT

It never hurts to plan ahead when you're not entirely sure where you'll dine out. Pack a to-go snack, toss it in your bag or car, and if you can't find something on the menu that's gluten friendly, you can munch on your backup snack instead.

In addition, a number of smartphone apps focus on gluten-free eating. There's no one-size-fits-all app—some focus on grocery shopping, while others highlight gluten-free restaurants—so check out a few before you need one. (See Appendix B for some apps we find helpful.)

Remember that ingredient lists might list only wheat-free options. Consider contacting the restaurant to learn more about the ingredients to ensure it's also gluten free and safe for you to eat.

Even when you do find some items you can eat on fast-food restaurant menus, remain vigilant. Don't assume those foods will always be gluten free. As with prepackaged foods, fast-food restaurants change their recipes occasionally, and sometimes they might swap a gluten-free filler for a wheat-based filler. In one small measure, the food that was once safe for you to eat has become unsafe. Check websites and ingredient lists often to be sure you catch any of these changes.

When you're visiting a fast-food restaurant, ask if they have a fryer dedicated to gluten-free foods. If not, those french fries could be ripe with cross-contamination. Discuss your concerns with the manager. Learn if there is a possibility of cross-contamination, and how it could be mitigated. For example, at Qdoba or Chipotle, just ask your food preparer to change gloves before he or she makes your burrito without the tortilla.

Some fast-food menu items may be premanufactured, or not made from scratch at the restaurant. You could order a burger without a bun to avoid gluten, but that premade burger could be mixed with a glutenous filler, and there's nothing you can do about it.

This all brings us back to an important point: the more whole foods you eat, the better your chances of not accidentally eating gluten in a processed food.

 GLUTEN GAFFE

> Avoid salad bars, buffets, and other serve-yourself restaurants where cross-contamination is just about guaranteed. That crouton spoon probably found its way to the iceberg lettuce bin at one point, or maybe the breaded chicken spatula was used to serve creamed corn. If you find yourself in such a place, ask to speak to the manager. Request that your food be served from the kitchen instead. Explain the concerns about cross-contamination so your food isn't contaminated in the kitchen.

Sample Different Cuisines

Many cuisines feature dishes that are specifically gluten-free. Others can easily be modified to be free of gluten, while others such as tabbouleh or couscous, which have gluten-based main ingredients, should be avoided.

You might encounter a language barrier in some restaurants. Always be polite when you explain your gluten-free diet, and if your server doesn't understand, ask to speak to the manager. If you still don't feel you're being understood, you might be on your own to find a suitable replacement. Look for green salads—minus the croutons—and make a mental note that the restaurant doesn't have much for you to eat.

When your food arrives, check it carefully before taking a bite. If you don't feel like you received definite confirmation that your request was understood and honored, don't eat the meal. Never, ever eat something just to be polite. The days of eating something you're not quite sure about are over. Don't be bullied or guilted into eating something you don't want to eat.

If you were clear in your order and the salad arrives with croutons, politely but firmly send it back. If you haven't touched it, you should be entitled to a gluten-free replacement without paying for a second dish.

When you visit a restaurant that focuses on a particular cuisine, you still need to probably avoid soups, marinades, dressings, and sauces because wheat-based thickeners or soy sauce may be used during preparation. Fried foods are frequently dipped in a wheat-based batter before frying. Instead, look for broiled or roasted meats and fresh, steamed, or boiled vegetables without sauces.

At Chinese restaurants, it's important that you confirm what's used in the cooking sauces. Besides using wheat as a thickener, some Chinese dishes contain wheat-filled soy sauce. Look instead for roasted, steamed, or broiled meats. Rice noodles or steamed vegetables may be easy options, too, but tread carefully.

On Japanese menus, try the edamame, which are boiled soybeans in their pods. Before you order, confirm that buckwheat noodles are 100 percent buckwheat. Soy sauce, which isn't gluten free, appears in many dips, sauces, and dressings, so ask about its inclusion in dishes you're not sure about. Tamari-style sauce is often—but not always—gluten free, so ask if you're ordering sushi or sashimi. Skip tempura and fried foods, and anything with miso, because barley might contaminate it.

In Middle Eastern cuisine, bulgur is the star of the tabbouleh show, so avoid that dish. Glutenous couscous and pita breads are also often on these and Greek food menus. Skip the gyros and falafel, unless the chef can guarantee they contain no wheat. Moussaka and spanokopita have wheat as a general ingredient, so take a pass on those, too. Good options are hummus or baba ghanoush and fresh vegetables. You should be able to eat souvlaki as well.

Dal and yogurt-based raita are excellent choices at Indian restaurants. Many of the breads are a miss, but papadums are made from lentils and should be a safe replacement. Dosa, which are generally made from a rice mixture, should be good to go, but do confirm with the chef before ordering. Meats are generally safe, such as Tandoori chicken. Skip the samosas, which are dough wrapped around fillings. If the restaurant serves pakora, you might ask about it being gluten free. But both samosas and pakora are fried and could present cross-contamination.

DEFINITION

Dal is generally a dried pea, bean, or legume used in Indian cooking. Some of the names you may run across in this staple of Indian cuisine are *urad, toovar, massor,* and *mung.*

When it comes to Italian food, most pasta is out—unless the restaurant specifically serves gluten-free pasta cooked in its own water. (This is happening more and more!) Although not all risottos contain cheese or cream, some of them do, so if you can tolerate lactose, risotto might be a good choice. Antipasto is a go, as are simple, grilled meats. If the restaurant has gluten-free pasta, it may also offer gluten-free crusts for pizza. Check the ingredients, if possible, and ask how it's prepared. You might want to request your pizza be cooked on an extra sheet of aluminum foil to avoid potential cross-contamination.

Traditionally speaking, most marinaras, bolognaise, and ragus should be gluten free. Carbonaras and Alfredo sauces, if they're made from scratch, should be fine, too. But if the Alfredo sauce isn't from scratch, chances are it contains gluten. Be sure to ask if the marinara and other tomato-based sauces are thickened with pasta water. If so, avoid them.

Polenta is corn-based, so as long as the accompanying sauce doesn't have gluten and isn't mixed with additional grains, you should be fine. You might think potato gnocchi is safe, but often some flour is mixed in. Clear soups may be possible, but avoid minestrone because it usually contains pasta. Avoid the bread basket and breadsticks. Ask the chef or your server about anything you're not sure about.

At Mexican restaurants, masa harina is the main ingredient in many fresh-baked corn tortillas, and thankfully, it's safe for gluten-free diners. Enchiladas are typically made with corn tortillas, but confirm before ordering. However, do ask if the corn chips are fried in a fryer that also fries other foods. If so, pass on the chips and salsa. Corn tamales should be okay, but ask about the preparation to ensure they're gluten free. Elizabeth has heard that some of the red or green sauces served with Mexican dishes are thickened with flours. Again, ask when you're not sure. Ceviche, which may appear on a menu at Spanish and Latin restaurants, is fish marinated in lime juice.

In French restaurants, you might think you should order everything plain, but if the chef makes certain sauces the traditional way, they should be naturally gluten free. Ask about such sauces as beurre blanc, hollandaise, béarnaise, sauce choron. If they're not made from scratch, some hollandaise and béarnaise sauces are thickened with wheat flour. Avoid béchamel sauce, mornay sauce, and many wine-based reductions in French restaurants. You also need to find out if any entrée ingredients have been dredged in flour. Some chefs dredge chicken breasts and fish fillets in flour before pan-frying.

Seafood restaurants serve a scampi sauce that's French inspired, and shrimp scampi, if it's traditionally cooked, is gluten free. But watch for breadcrumbs sprinkled on top of the shrimp. Sometimes it's served over wheat noodles, so be sure to ask before ordering.

Eating with Friends

Humans are social creatures, and there likely will come a time when you're invited to a friend's dinner party. Your first thought upon receiving the invitation is, *What will I eat?* That's normal.

As a lifelong food-allergy sufferer, Elizabeth has had a lot of practice calling friends, thanking them for the party invitation, and asking if she can bring anything. She follows this with, "Oh, and, by the way, my family doesn't eat gluten. I'm not sure what you plan to serve, but will that be okay?" Keep it casual and polite, and you'll start the conversation on the right foot.

Explain what gluten is, give the host an idea of some foods that contain gluten, and ask about the menu. Together, the two of you can determine if the meal plan works for you. Lasagna and Italian bread? Probably not. Roast chicken and mashed potatoes? Sounds good! If you can't reach an agreement, or you don't want to inconvenience your host, you can volunteer to bring something to contribute that's safe for you to eat, or you can eat before you go.

 TASTY TIDBIT

If you bring your own food, still be wary of cross-contamination, especially if your food will be cooked alongside glutenous foods. For example, if you're invited to a cookout, bring your own hamburger or gluten-free hot dog wrapped in aluminum foil so it doesn't come into contact with any gluten—and to make it easier on your host.

Social situations often are more about the socializing and less about the surrounding elements. Enjoy your friends and family without making a big deal about your gluten-free eating. By bringing your own items, you'll show you're serious about avoiding gluten but still interested in socializing.

Gluten-Free Travel

Travel is often fraught with uncertainty, even if you aren't gluten free. But with a little research and advance planning, you can hit the road without worrying about possible gluten encounters.

It's immensely helpful if you can bring a few safe items to eat, just in case you're hungry and stuck in a glutenous zone.

Plan Ahead

Before you pack a suitcase, you should make some arrangements so you can travel more easily as a gluten-free eater.

On a road trip, for example, you might want to study your route to determine where you can stop to eat or load up on snacks. If you see a sea of gas stations between your home and your destination, cook some extra meals before you leave, pack a cooler, and eat like a king along the way. Otherwise, you may be stuck eating sunflower seeds and gluten-free beef jerky.

Are there fast-food restaurants along the way? If so, check out their websites to find gluten-free options. If you're going to visit friends or family, ask for recommendations of places to stop. But still do your own research about the gluten-free offerings, too. Your diet is yours, and they may not understand what is involved.

 TASTY TIDBIT

For a directory of restaurants that offer specialized foods or meals, check out *ViVa's Healthy Dining Guide* by Lisa Margolin and Connie Dee. It lists 2,100 healthy dining options across the United States.

Heading to a resort or hotel, or going on a cruise? Call ahead to request special meals. Some tour companies, hotels, and resorts provide gluten-free options. But plan on re-confirming as the dates near for your trip. Starting an open dialogue and getting a helpful person's name goes a long way to ensure someone at your destination knows your concerns.

In recent years, a few hotel chains have started catering to the concerns of the gluten-free traveler, at least in the United States. As of this writing, Marriott, Hyatt, Hilton, and Carlson hotels are gluten aware. More might be by the time you read this. Check glutenfreehotelsguide.com to see if your hotel offers gluten-free options.

Also, consider requesting a room with a kitchen so you can prepare your own food. In fact, for the most flexibility, that might help you determine where to stay.

If you're staying at a bed and breakfast on your trip, call ahead to discuss your dietary needs.

Many cruise lines cater to gluten-free travelers. Holland America, for example, has one chef on each ship whose sole responsibility is cooking for people who are gluten free, suffer from allergies, or have other dietary concerns. If you're going on a cruise, contact your ship at least 2 weeks before your scheduled departure to be sure they're aware of your needs.

It's important to remember that this one chef works for the main dining room and specialty restaurants on the ship, not the regular buffet. The buffet chefs might be able to safely get you a gluten-free muffin to go with your scrambled eggs or a gluten-free cookie to go with your salad, but they might put your gluten-free bread in the regular toaster if you don't tell them not to.

If you still feel uncertain, investigate gluten-free tour groups. If you're with others who understand your plight, you might find yourself actually relaxing and enjoying your trip, rather than worrying about where you're going to eat your next meal. Request to speak to one of the group's previous travelers, if you can, to ensure it's the right group for you before you book.

The Gluten-Free-Friendly Skies

Elizabeth was traveling recently and was pleasantly surprised at some of the gluten-free options available in airports and on airlines. In the Denver International Airport, for example, Udi's Café and Bar, operated by a Colorado-based bakery, provides gluten-free options for travelers.

If you know what airport you're flying into, do a little research. Many airports have websites where they list the restaurants and other businesses in the terminal. Even if you don't know what terminal you're flying into, you can still get an idea of some places where you can eat.

Fast food is one option, but don't assume double fryers is a given, as it might be in other fast-food places. Avoid fried foods to reduce your risk of cross-contamination.

Many airlines are happy to oblige your diet, but in Elizabeth's experience, gluten-free meals aren't always one of the standard dietary options. Getting a gluten-free alternative involves a phone call to the airlines. This is also a good way to find out if the airline you're traveling even offers a gluten-free menu.

 GLUTEN GAFFE

Some airlines don't provide a gluten-free snack or meal option if the flight is less than 4 hours long.

If possible, give airlines at least 72 hours to plan for your gluten-free request. But always pack some extra food in reusable containers just in case, even if it's a short flight. Your flight could get delayed, and you could be stuck on a plane where the only snack options are pretzels. Don't forget to fill up for your return trip, too.

Packing Food

It would be nice if you didn't have to bring your own food when you travel, but it's still a good idea. Even with all your researching and plans, you might run into a problem on the road. Maybe the resort only offers a gluten-free breakfast option, or the meal plan is for two meals a day and you need to find alternatives for a third meal. Whatever it is, you'll feel better if you have some safe food with you to eat.

Even when Elizabeth visits family, she packs extra food. Her siblings are not gluten-free, so she tries to plan accordingly and pack some foods to last until she can visit the grocery store.

If you're staying in a place with a mini-kitchen, pack gluten-free pasta. If you're going to be touring and are unsure of your options, pack gluten-free snack bars (homemade or purchased). Include enough for each day … and then add extras. You just never know.

If you run out of your standbys, find a grocery store and see if you can purchase some gluten-free options there.

If You Accidentally Eat Gluten

Unfortunately, unless you're allergic to wheat, there's nothing you can take to alleviate your symptoms if you accidentally consume gluten. If you're allergic, you may experience a histamine reaction, which will respond to an antihistamine. Some gluten-intolerant folks don't even have a noticeable reaction. If you do, here are some suggestions for coping.

First, it might help to know you're not alone. Others have been where you are, and you will get through this.

With a peanut allergy and gluten intolerance, Elizabeth has learned that panic rarely solves a problem, but it *can* exacerbate a situation. Even though you aren't at home, you should take a deep breath and try to assess what's happened and what your options are. Can you break away from the group activities to rest and recuperate? Perhaps you can find a quiet place to rest, feel better, and rejoin your group later.

Once your reaction has subsided, trace your steps to figure out where the contamination occurred. If it's a place where you'll have to visit again, determine what you can do to ensure it doesn't happen again. Do you or your travel group need to speak with a manager? Or can you avoid that location for the rest of the trip? If not, what can you do differently next time?

 FOOD FOR THOUGHT

Currently, there are many debates about what you can do or take to minimize the damage when you've ingested gluten. Some suggest vomiting, while others suggest taking a probiotic with lots of water. Still others recommend digestive enzymes that can help minimize any gluten slips and any inflammation caused by the slip. Consult with your health-care provider to decide what's best for you.

The Least You Need to Know

- Plan for eating out at restaurants, and research what you can eat beforehand— even call to confirm during nonpeak meal times.

- Gluten-free fast-food options exist, but investigate them thoroughly before you take your first bite.

- Research and plan for any trip. But always pack extra gluten-free food with you as well.

- Before you accidentally ingest gluten, talk to your health-care provider to find out the best course of treatment should you slip.

CHAPTER 10

Gluten-Free Entertaining

When you realized you needed to give up gluten, one of the first questions you might have asked yourself is, *How will I ever feel normal again?* Being the social creatures we are, eating with friends and family can help maintain and restore feelings of normalcy. After all, food is often central to our socializing. We go out to dinner. We stop by for coffee. We meet for drinks.

The safest way to avoid gluten at dinners and parties is to host the festivities yourself and provide a delicious and nutritious gluten-free spread for your guests to enjoy. You've probably played the host before, in your glutenous days. The premise is the same now. You might need to do a bit more planning, but we show you how in this chapter.

Also, be prepared to talk about your gluten-free way of eating at the gathering. Folks will enjoy your food so much, you're sure to receive compliments and requests for recipes. So plan a few responses in advance so you'll feel comfortable talking about why you're avoiding gluten.

In This Chapter

- Hosting a gluten-free party
- Planning your menu
- Surviving pitch-ins
- Imbibing without suffering

Of course, for many, a party isn't complete without alcohol. Beers, generally, are off limits on a gluten-free diet. But what about alcohol made with grain and the mixers you may encounter? We go over the ins and outs of imbibing in this chapter, too.

Planning a Party

By now, your friends and family probably know you're eating gluten free. So why not throw a gluten-free soirée to show them some of the wonderful foods you're enjoying now?

Because you're in charge, this should be fairly easy to handle, with some planning.

Start Small

The easiest part of hosting your own gluten-free party or holiday get-together is using foods you've made and know are delicious and especially gluten free. We suggest starting with a small dinner party of close friends or family who know about your gluten-intolerance. (A big, blowout party may include friends of friends who are less aware you're gluten free. Wait to host the big party or holiday gathering until a few months down the line.)

Begin removing the gluten from the very beginning of your planning, starting with the invites. As you call or email your potential guests, explain the idea behind your party, spell out why you're eating gluten free now, and emphasize your guests don't need to bring anything food-wise with them. This gets the gluten-free thought in their head early and ensures you don't accidently receive a thank you gift of a loaf of homemade glutenous bread.

At the party, you want to ensure your guests understand the rules of your gluten-free kitchen. That may sound uncomfortable and unfestive, but it's necessary. We're not suggesting you invite friends and family into your home and then have them sign on the dotted line that they've read and accept your house rules. But letting people know early about your gluten intolerance helps everyone manage better.

No matter how small you start, you'll still probably be nervous about feeding your friends gluten-free foods. That's normal. Just fix some of your favorites and know they may not know what to expect either.

 FOOD FOR THOUGHT

Reportedly, one third of the American population lives with some kind of food sensitivity. Wheat is one of eight main allergens. So you might not be the only person at your gathering with a food intolerance.

We wish we had a dollar for each time we've heard, "How can you eat gluten free?" or "I tried gluten-free bread once, and it was horrible. I could never eat gluten free." Some of your friends may even respond the same way, so for your first party, don't invite anyone you think will be anything less than supportive of your food.

If anyone does remark about the pasta or bread tasting different, don't get defensive. Patiently explain your new diet and why the difference in taste.

Prepare the Zone for Guests

If your kitchen has areas for gluten and nongluten foods, we suggest you create a sign to indicate the gluten free zone with a request that "If you have a question, please ask!"

Why a sign? Two reasons: it can help explain your two sets of utensils and serving spoons, and a sign is a way of announcing the change, which can lead to discussion, not defensiveness. Making the sign playful and fun or artful and pretty can put your guests more at ease.

This might seem like overkill, but we've found it's a good ice-breaker. Your guests will be curious, and it's easier to explain the gluten-free zones than to point out when a guest has accidentally contaminated the gluten-free area.

 TASTY TIDBIT

If you don't feel artistic enough to create a sign, companies that specialize in gluten-free kitchen gear, such as gluten-free serving spoons by The Food Allergy Kitchen-ware Co. (foodallergykitchenware.com) or CafePress (cafepress.com), sell stickers and magnets to ensure your gluten-free zone is visible.

You may have already conquered making a clear gluten-free zone when you were setting up your kitchen. If the kitchen is completely gluten free, it'll be easier to see when someone brings a loaf of glutenous bread and inadvertently violates your gluten-free kitchen.

When this happens, thank your guest for bringing something, but mention you need to keep everything free of gluten. This opens the door for a discussion of gluten, why you have to avoid it, and how even the smallest amount can make you sick. But do so in a nice and polite way so you don't make your thoughtful guest feel bad for bringing the wrong thing.

If someone does bring some bread or other glutenous item, wait until they're out of the kitchen, and do a quick cleanup of the area. If you have a gluten-free kitchen with a solitary sponge, don't contaminate it. Instead, use paper towels and cleaning solution to disinfect the area and clear out the gluten.

Don't Invite Gluten

When having friends over, it helps to plan a menu that doesn't depend on or hint at the need for bread or other foods that contain gluten. Don't even provide for the opportunity to invite gluten to your party.

The standard American diet frequently features glutenous foods. How many spaghetti dinners have you been to, for example, that included garlic or Italian bread? Even if you're preparing gluten-free pasta, a guest may bring his or her "favorite bread for pasta dinners."

Work to plan a meal without a gluten component. For *hors d'oeuvres,* serve cheeses, fruits, and homemade Gluten-Free Crackers or Chickpea Flatbread (Chapter 18). Choose an entrée of Arroz con Pollo (Chapter 16) or a roast chicken with mashed potatoes and broccoli on the side. (Even if you make a gravy for the potatoes, you can use a gluten-free thickener like arrowroot.) If you're planning on grilling, try a piece of salmon served with rice and asparagus. Dessert can come in all shapes and sizes—check out Chapter 19 for yummy ideas.

Party Planning Pointers

One of the best ways to have fun at your party is to keep it simple. Don't prepare two meals—one for you and one for friends who can eat gluten. You'll double your work, and the more work you do hosting, the less fun you'll have. Instead, create one awesome gluten-free meal, including a delectable dessert, that's sure to earn you (and gluten-free foods) rave reviews.

Also, make the dishes you plan to serve a couple times at other meals before you invite everyone over to try them. Don't make your party the first time you cook the dishes.

Plan for Success

When she was young, Elizabeth remembers watching her mother plan for a party, making a guest list, a menu list, and a grocery list. That advance planning takes a bit of time at the beginning but lets you check things off your lists as you go and can help reduce your stress level because you don't have to worry about whether you forgot something or someone. So get your pen and paper, and let's make some lists.

 FOOD FOR THOUGHT

The first list Elizabeth makes is one detailing a meal she feels sure she can pull off. There's nothing like preparing chicken biryani for the first time and miscalculating how long it takes to prepare—which might have happened before Elizabeth started making lists. Luckily, the dinner party she hosted included close friends and the conversation flowed. But obviously, that was the last time Elizabeth winged it.

As you become more familiar with gluten-free cooking, you'll begin to master your own meals. After all, food is now more than something to socialize around. Meals can be healing for you.

Keep notes in your food diary about what herbs or spices went well with what. Also note what meals you liked and which ones to not make again. For the holidays, Elizabeth makes a pie to which she's added and subtracted ingredients to suit her family's tastes. Also, start planning meals with more whole foods than processed foods.

But if something does go wrong with the cooking (like biryani taking too long to cook), keep your sense of humor. Continue to smile and be a gracious host. Instead of fretting over the misstep, enjoy your extra time to socialize with your guests. As long as you maintain your cool, no one will know it's not as perfect as you envisioned it ... unless you have a grease fire with your tortilla Espanola, which is what happened to Jeanette. Her husband, who she wasn't even dating at the time, was a guest and was impressed at her making a meal from scratch. But when they did start dating, the first gift he bought her was a fire extinguisher.

Menu Planning

Elizabeth likes to determine in advance what she's going to prepare because this helps her plan the theme of her party. For example, are your Lemon Poppy Seed Scones (Chapter 18) incredibly moist and delicious? Or have you found a delectable gluten-free coffee cake or Sausage, Cheese, and Spinach Breakfast Casserole (Chapter 13)? You might want to fix one of these items for a brunch, alongside a fruit salad and glasses of sparkling wine and orange juice mimosas.

Once you've decided your menu, you can determine your guest list. When Elizabeth plans her meal first, she has a better idea of how many people she can invite. If you want to start with your guest list, that's okay, too.

For a hearty brisket, you need to have an idea of how many people you can feed from the recipe. If you decide to make a gluten-free jambalaya, you need to know if the recipe feeds six to eight or four to six.

We can't stress enough that you should invite a handful of people who will be supportive of your new diet and lifestyle. Plan your guest list carefully, and remember, this is just one of many gluten-free events you'll host. As your level of confidence in cooking gluten free grows, you'll feel more comfortable inviting larger groups of friends and family.

 TASTY TIDBIT

As you deliver your party invitations, ask your guests if they have any food allergies or intolerances you should know about. By extending this courtesy, they'll be more likely to remember you have food sensitivities, and you can start the conversation rolling.

When shopping for your ingredients, buy the freshest, highest-quality, whole foods possible. Higher-quality food tastes better, which is definitely one of the key concepts for a dinner party.

Also opt for ingredients easy to find during the season you're preparing the meal. Maybe February isn't the month to prepare sautéed zucchini if zucchini isn't in season in the winter months where you live. If, however, oranges are in season in February where you live, the Cranberry Orange Muffins in Chapter 18 might be perfect.

Anyone for Potluck?

When you're invited to a pitch-in, you don't have as much control over the foods and ingredients. Navigating a potluck can be tricky, so take a few precautions to ensure you avoid gluten. It's essential that you plan ahead and come prepared.

Don't just roll the dice when venturing to a potluck. It's your responsibility to be sure you don't accidentally get any gluten on your plate.

Bring Something You Can Eat

It might seem obvious to bring something to a pitch-in you know you can eat, but think about how many times you've been invited to a potluck and asked to bring a certain dish. Maybe the host asks you to make a salad or a dessert, for example. That might have been fine when you could eat anything, but now that you're gluten free, you need to look out for yourself.

You need to be able to bring an entrée, not just a side dish. After all, if you're going to enjoy yourself—and not be hungry throughout the party—your fruit salad can't be the only safe food there. Bring a dish you can eat. If there's nothing else safe for you, at least you have your go-to food.

If you can't bring an entrée, either eat before you attend the party or bring an entrée for yourself. If everyone is diving into the lasagna, who's going to notice you're eating a piece of chicken? And if someone does, chances are they won't see your chicken as contraband. It's a potluck, after all.

 GLUTEN GAFFE

Don't assume the menu will be gluten-free just because it has been in the past. Jeanette made that mistake at a family barbecue when she thought her aunt would make hamburgers and sausage links. Instead, the entrées were fried chicken and pulled pork, and the salads were ramen noodles and pasta salad. All Jeanette could eat was potato chips and fruit salad.

Elizabeth married into a big party-planning family with a growing and shifting multitude of dietary restrictions. Over the years, communally prepared holiday or vacation meals have given way to potluck extravaganzas. If someone prepares a gluten-free taco salad, great. If not, you can eat what you brought or your own gluten-free contraband.

Even if you bring your own dish, be careful about cross-contamination of serving utensils. If someone has used the knife to cut bread and then used the same knife for the butter spread, avoid using that spread on your own gluten-free bread you brought. Place your gluten-free food away from where someone might use your serving spoon to serve spaghetti or tabbouleh salad.

Organize Out the Gluten

We live in a digital world. So when planning your gluten-free party, don't forget to use some of the technological tools available.

A few years ago, when Elizabeth's in-laws were planning an annual get together, some of the grandchildren recognized the food restrictions and hurdles when considering menu planning for nearly 50 people. They created and shared a Google Drive document and used it to keep track of the vegetarians and peanut-, gluten-, and lactose-free relatives. It became a reference to help plan meals.

You can do something similar to ensure your potluck's ratio of desserts to dinner foods isn't too skewed in one direction or another.

If you're not strong on the technology or you prefer to speak with your guests beforehand, when you invite them, mention your celiac disease and what you plan to serve. You can use this time to ask them about any ingredients they have trouble with, too. Then, you can add notes to your guest list next to the names of any folks who have a food issue. When you're making your grocery list, keep track of what ingredients your guests have trouble with and accommodate as much as possible.

Once you take charge of what people are bringing, and especially what they're not bringing (gluten), you'll breathe easier and can focus on making the event a success.

What About Alcohol?

Approach drinking alcohol with caution because certain alcohols and most beers contain a glutenous grain during their production. Conduct your research long before you head to the liquor store to buy booze for your party. Learn what each type of alcohol is made from so you won't be surprised.

Choose Carefully

In theory, all distilled alcohol should be gluten-free because the distillation process removes the gluten proteins. For example, scotch distilleries process their alcohol using wheat, rye, or barley. Distilling the grains removes the gluten, so the general consensus is that distilled alcohol should be okay. In fact, the Canadian Celiac Association says that "since they are distilled, they do not contain prolamins [gluten proteins] and are allowed unless otherwise indicated." But the Celiac Sprue Association doesn't agree.

Distillation, if done properly, should remove all the gluten, but not all spirits manufacturers actually distill properly so their vodka or gins or ryes or whatever may still contain gluten. Some distillers add a grain mash during the final process, so gluten could be returned to a distilled alcohol.

Do you have a favorite alcohol? If so, check out the manufacturer's website. You might even call the company to discuss its process. If it mentions adding some mash as part of the post-distillation finishing process, ask what grain is used. The distilled alcohol may not be a problem, but the additional grain may be.

Beer is a clear miss at parties because its main ingredient is malted barley or another glutenous grain. The hops used in beer are gluten free.

You don't need to be a party pooper, but do avoid alcohols or mixers that add colors, flavors, or additives because they may contain gluten. If you do use mixers, read the labels carefully and avoid mixers that contain gluten.

Gluten-Free Alcohol

Gluten-free alcohols occupy many shelves at the liquor store. Some have even received the right to display gluten-free labels. Blue Ice Vodka, for example, is a potato vodka produced in Idaho and was the first to receive the right to label its product gluten free. The Alcohol and Tobacco Tax and Trade Bureau, which oversees alcohol labeling, bestowed this labeling right in April 2013.

But watch out, because not all vodka brands are gluten free and some are made from rye or wheat. Instead, you might want to drink one of the following:

- Wines, including champagne; brandy; and other grape-based drinks
- Rum, made from sugar cane
- Tequila, made from the agave plant
- Gin (when made from potatoes)

Wine is a safe bet. Brandy, because it's distilled from wine, is safe, as is grappa, also made from grapes.

But although wine is a safe bet, wine coolers are not. Many wine coolers are made with malted barley, which contains gluten. If you prefer a sweeter and effervescent wine product, try sangria, made with sparkling wine. Or make your own wine coolers with wine and sparkling water or club soda. Add a refreshing splash of your favorite fruit juice.

If liquor or wine are not your style, explore gluten-free beers. The market is expanding, and many brewers are producing beers made with gluten-free ingredients like buckwheat, corn, millet, rice, or sorghum.

In 2006, Lakefront Brewery of Milwaukee convinced the federal government to allow them to produce beer made from sorghum instead of malted barley. Previously, federal regulation required beer to be made from one-quarter malted barley. Lakefront Brewery became the first American brewery to make a gluten-free beer.

Spanish Estrella Damm Daura is an award-winning gluten-free beer made from malted barley, hops, and pearl rice. Not only does the manufacturer make the beer using barley, it also tests the beer to ensure it falls far below the 20 parts per million (ppm) of allowed gluten. According to its website, Estrella Damm Daura tests at 3 ppm, well below the 20 ppm.

FOOD FOR THOUGHT

The gluten-free beer business is booming. Some of the different kinds available—with varying price tags and nationalities—are Bard's, St. Peter's, Dogfish Head Tweason Ale, Redbridge, Green's, New Planet, New Grist, Estrella Damm Daura, and Omission. Also check out the Gluten-Free Beer app to help you decide what to pour into your frosty mug. Online, you can find a top 10 list of gluten-free beers at bonappetit.com/blogsandforums/blogs/badaily/2013/02/gluten-free-beer-tastes-good.html.

The Least You Need to Know

- Especially when you're just starting out, plan small get-togethers with close friends who will support your gluten-free eating style.
- Make lists to help you keep track of the menu, what you need to get at the grocery store, and the guests you plan on inviting along with any of their allergy or intolerance problems.
- You can host and enjoy a party—even if you drink alcohol; you just need some careful planning and vigilance.

CHAPTER 11

Gluten-Free Kids

If you have celiac disease, the odds increase that your children will also develop gluten intolerance because celiac disease strikes at the genetic level. When you have a child, keeping him in a gluten-free zone can be challenging, particularly if he doesn't show any symptoms.

In keeping your child safe outside your home, depending on the age of your child, one of the first lines of defense is his school or caregiver. Helping his teacher and other adults understand what your child needs gives him another safe place.

Of course, birthday parties—pizza and cake anyone?—are one of the major childhood events every parent of a gluten-intolerant child faces (dreads?). Our suggestions in this chapter should help you and your children cope with common situations, ranging from early ages to college.

In This Chapter

* Keeping your child free of gluten
* Working with teachers and other caregivers
* Navigating birthdays and other parties
* The gluten-free teen and young adult

Keeping Caregivers and Teachers Informed

For years of your child's life, teachers or caregivers of some sort will see him many hours a day. Establishing a rapport with these adults benefits you and your child—educationally as well as with any dietary issues.

Let's Talk About It

At some point, no matter your parenting style, you'll need to leave your child with a relative, a babysitter, a day-care center, or a school. If he's gluten sensitive, you'll need to communicate this condition with others.

At the same time, you'll also need to start teaching your child about the food choices he should and shouldn't make. You can never start too early to educate your child and his caregivers.

 TASTY TIDBIT

Don't approach the school administrators, nurses, or teachers as adversaries. Always be polite and professional. Schedule a meeting to discuss your gluten-intolerant child and the best way you all can work together to support his dietary challenge.

Just as you enter discussions with friends, your approach with a caregiver should be similar. Be clear and concise about your child's situation.

If a babysitter is coming into your home to care for your child, make that person aware of any allergies or concerns. But especially if the sitting occurs outside the home, put your child's needs in writing. Talking about them might not be enough.

Put It in Writing

Vigilance is the name of the game here. Put the information about your child's gluten sensitivities in as many places as possible. Whether you type a letter or fill out a form in ink, be sure your caregivers understand your child's health situation. Leave detailed instructions on the care of your gluten-intolerant child in as many places as you can because, even with the most trusted babysitter, you may run into issues.

Elizabeth's encounter with a trusted babysitter—so trusted the babysitting took place outside the family home—still guides how she dispels information to caregivers. She learned the hard way and often replays in her head returning home and seeing her child walking toward her still holding the offending food and reacting to the gluten in it. What happened? The babysitter thought a particular food was okay. Without a written list, she had no way to double-check, and she didn't want to bother Elizabeth in her meeting. Lesson learned.

Elizabeth's encounter helped confirm that, even with the best babysitters and family members, it's essential that she explain in detail what foods are okay and what foods are off-limits. She's also learned to make a list and review it with the caregiver before she leaves.

You must really spell it out like this. Take any and all guesswork completely out of the picture, and be sure your child's caregivers understand the seriousness of the situation.

In the Classroom

At the beginning of each school year, schools provide a stack of paperwork for parents to fill out. Be sure you complete these papers carefully.

In addition to the aforementioned annual papers, each time your child goes on a field trip, you receive another form, a permission slip. This is another opportunity for you to let the school know of your child's food challenges.

But don't leave it at the paper level. Be proactive by looking for ways you can reach out to administrators so they better understand your child's illness. For example, get involved in your child's schooling by offering to help during art, at parties, or on field trips. This helps engender a familiarity that allows conversations to naturally occur with school administration, nurses, teachers, and aides.

In a school setting, maybe you feel comfortable packing your child a lunch or other food each day. For a younger child, you might feel more comfortable approaching the classroom teacher or school administrators to explain and offer: "My child has an allergy to wheat. I'd like to bring in wheat-free food he can eat at the same time his classmates have their morning snacks."

You may even want to start a discussion with the food preparers: "My child has celiac disease/gluten intolerance/a wheat allergy, which means he cannot eat anything with gluten in it. Can we please review how you prepare food in the kitchen? I'd like to see if we could work on a plan to prevent cross-contamination."

But be sure school personnel understand there's no medicine a gluten-intolerant person can take to get better, and eating a gluten-free diet is the prescribed method for dealing with this health situation. Provide the school with a copy of the doctor's written prescription for your child's gluten-free diet. Make extra copies in case you need them for other authorities, but keep the original filed safely away.

If the child has a wheat allergy and the reaction is different from those with an intolerance, also provide the school with your child's prescribed antihistamine or epinephrine pen.

The U.S. government recognizes the need for accommodations for a diagnosed gluten-free child. (You may suspect your child has food issues, but you'll need the written diagnosis from the child's doctor.) If your child's school participates in the federal lunch food program and your child has received a doctor's "prescription" for this diet, you, as a parent, are not *required* to provide a gluten-free option. According to the federal program, schools that prepare foods must buy gluten-free options from a commercial source. (You could still approach the school's food preparers with your concerns, as noted earlier.)

What if your child attends a private school that doesn't participate in the federal lunch program but does provide lunch? As long as your child has a doctor's prescription for a gluten-free diet, the private school must make accommodations.

The law in question is Section 504 of the Rehabilitation Act of 1973, which forbids the discrimination of anyone on the basis of a disability in an educational program or institution. Celiac is considered a disability and is now covered within this federal statute.

FOOD FOR THOUGHT

If your child attends a school that participates in the National School Lunch Program, you are not required to provide gluten-free options for the school's kitchen. If your child attends a private school with a food program, the Americans with Disabilities Act mandates that your child's medically prescribed gluten-free diet is covered and needs to be accommodated.

For more information on navigating the school system, and for suggested letters and 504 plan outlines, log on to the National Foundation for Celiac Awareness's website (celiaccentral.org/kids/parents/guides/Kids-Youth/Navigating-The-School-System/209).

Regardless of how many notes and forms you fill out, you'll still need to politely and respectfully discuss gluten intolerance with your child's teachers and administrators. In the long run, you might find it better for your child to bring a packed lunch.

Kid Reminders

Don't rely only on your communication with caregivers and teachers. Also teach your child:

- Teach him to ask about ingredients.
- Show him how to refuse food politely.
- Give him options for coping with not always getting to eat what everyone else gets to eat.

For a younger child, consider investing in an allergy bracelet. Elizabeth bought a fun-looking food allergy bracelet—for three years and older—that comes with the standard eight allergens—peanut, shellfish, wheat, soy, dairy, fish, tree nuts, and eggs—which can be mixed and matched.

Medical charms can be added to the bracelet, too, for gluten or strawberry allergies, among others.

Such a bracelet can help make your child aware, but we suggest he wear it only when going to an event, which makes his aware that others need to know of his allergy.

> **GLUTEN GAFFE**
>
> Even with all these precautions, a gluten-intolerant child could still manage to share food with a friend or be given a "treat" that causes a problem. If this happens, take a deep breath, explain, and keep educating others about your child's condition.

You might give your child a preprinted business card explaining his dietary needs he can hand to the cafeteria staff each day. It can become part of the daily routine so the lunch staff understands the importance of being vigilant on behalf of your child—not just some days, but *every* day.

Don't forget the great power of talking. Spend time at meals discussing foods and food awareness. Listen to your child's concerns and understanding of the gluten intolerance. Remember, a child's understanding differs from your own, so explain in age-appropriate language while supporting your child's belief in his own self and growth.

As your child ages, have him help you prepare meals and snack foods. Not only can this provide a bonding experience, but it also helps him become more aware of the use of different ingredients. It can also be educational as you add numbers, counting, and fractions. Cooking with your child also increases his palate for good foods. Jeanette has been cooking with her son since he was barely 1 year old. Today, he's the only 3-year-old she knows who loves kale and kalamata olives.

Teach your child to read labels and recognize safe foods. This is one way to start teaching him about the daily elements of gluten-free eating. Reading labels is also good for helping develop better literacy.

Just as you communicate with caregivers, keep the conversation going with your child. Explain—and get your health-care provider to help explain—what he needs to do to eat and live gluten free.

Coping with Celebrations

During the school year, celebrations seem to lurk around every corner. Whether it's a holiday party or a birthday party, kids love to celebrate, and so do their caregivers. Often events are planned around food and food activities—cookie decorating or a hundred pieces of candy for the hundredth day of school.

But to ensure your gluten-intolerant child enjoys the parties and doesn't end up ill, you might want to take a few preparations.

Prepping for School Parties

School policies often have a few lines about school celebrations. Read the policy closely to see how it impacts your child's classroom.

At one of the schools Elizabeth's children attended, each week teachers ordered an outside treat for their classes—pizza one week, sandwiches the next, for example. Parents would pay out-of-pocket for these treats, but the organizing parent would choose the restaurant.

Elizabeth's kids loved the program … except when everyone else would be eating a slice of cheese or pepperoni pizza and her children would be eating a cold sandwich from home. Some weeks, a gluten-free option would be available, but for the most part, that wasn't the case. Then, midway through the year, the school had to modify the program. Health department rules kicked in, and only certain food providers could deliver the food to the school. That narrowed the gluten-free options for Elizabeth's kids.

The point is, your county or city's health department rules can restrict what can be brought into schools, but that doesn't mean it will prevent allergens from arriving in the classroom.

 FOOD FOR THOUGHT

Your school district and schools probably receive their food policies from the area health department. Investigate your school's policy and the city or county's health department policy to better understand if homemade foods are allowed in classrooms or if only commercially produced food is allowed.

If this is the case in your child's school, you might want to enlist the help of his teacher and request that special treats be kept on hand for him. So if a classmate brings in doughnuts, for example, your child will have something special to eat as well. Does this idea work? Not always. Your child might still try the doughnut (or other glutenous food). But that becomes a moment to review the gluten-free rules and teach him how to be safe. For asymptomatic children, this can be a difficult lesson to learn.

Also, even though you want to bring in a homemade goodie, you might have to opt for a store-bought gluten-free one. The health department's rule about commercially prepared food might also restrict you bringing in homemade goods. Check with the school administration to see how that regulation works.

You also could meet with the parents of other allergic children—either within your child's grade or within the school. Discuss with them how they navigate the school's rules to support their own children.

If you've discussed the gluten-free necessity of your child with the school's administration and nurse, always follow up with a letter and track the responses you receive from the school. If, for whatever reason, you don't get support from the school personnel, the letters will be useful for you to review. At some point, it might become necessary to change schools.

Planning Gluten-Free Birthday Parties

When making plans for a gluten-free birthday party, consider finding a place where you can bring in your own food or a place that will accommodate your child's celiac disease. In Elizabeth's experience, many party options, unfortunately, offer a choice of pizzas and soda fountain drinks alongside a bring-your-own cake.

You'll need to employ some creativity:

- Don't plan a party around meal times.

- Make a gluten-free cake a week or two before the party to ensure your kids like the recipe, or serve it at a family-only party as a test.

- Schedule the party at a museum or garden or gymnastics center that doesn't normally have food facilities and may allow more flexibility in what foods you can bring.

- Rent a picnic shelter at a local park. Barbecuing may be an option, but if not, supply fresh vegetables and fruits.

Be sure to ask the parents of the children you're inviting if they have allergy concerns with their children before finalizing your menu.

A friend of Elizabeth's has a child with myriad allergies—eggs, soy, and certain nuts. A birthday party at Elizabeth's could be a relief for the mother and the one place—of only a few—the friend felt comfortable letting her son eat cake. Elizabeth always tries to make a point to ask what foods might be an issue. Also, because she often cooks with almond flour, she definitely doesn't want an allergic guest to feel left out at her home.

Attending a Non-Gluten-Free Birthday Party

When a friend or classmate invites your child to a birthday party, use some of the same techniques you use when a friend of yours invites you.

Many parties are scheduled through electronic invitations, but we encourage you to call the hosts to RSVP. That way, you can start the conversation about gifts for the child. Before you hang up, mention that your son or daughter has celiac disease and cannot ingest wheat: "Do you mind if I bring a special gluten-free cupcake for my child? I'd hate for him to miss out on Trudy's party and the celebration. I could bring a few extra cupcakes, if that would help calm any hurt feelings."

Always offer to bring extra. When you make the offer, ask if the birthday child has any allergies or food concerns.

You might even add baking to the list of activities you engage in with your child before attending a party: "Before we go buy Trevor a birthday present, we need to bake you a special treat for Trevor's party. Do you want to bring a chocolate or vanilla cupcake?" Then allow your child to help make the cupcakes. Remember, he'll more readily eat food he's helped make. If you don't bake, have him pick out a special store-bought treat. (Gluten-free rice treats are always a big hit.)

 TASTY TIDBIT

You probably already carry a stash of gluten-free food around for your own daily living. When it comes to special celebrations, prepare gluten-free party treats ahead of time—cupcakes or doughnuts—and freeze them for enjoying the day of the party.

But when attending a birthday party, always bring something special that's gluten free for your child. You don't want to make the treat stand out from what's being served, but just be sure it's something he enjoys. If you're planning the party for a nonceliac sibling, try to create a theme cake that allows for a gluten-free version as well, or just make one delicious gluten-free cake that no one recognizes as such. (We won't tell if you don't.)

Birthday cake is the obvious gluten in the party room, but check with the host about any other foods with hidden gluten, too. Here are a few suggestions where you might find gluten at a birthday party:

- Candy fallen from a piñata or given in treat bags—beware of the party candy

- Prepackaged drinks—perhaps a malted milkshake or flavored milk—check the labels, just in case

- Hot dogs and beans—some brands use wheat-based filler or barley coloring

Gluten and Older Children

Having to skip eating pizza can be difficult for a kid and even more so for a teen moving toward independence. Food is something he should be able to control, during a time when nearly everything seems out of control. But if he's gluten intolerant, he can't even have a say in that.

Getting teens and college students the resources they need can help them transition into supporting their own healthy gluten-free diet and lifestyle.

Celiac Teens

Most teenagers just want to fit in. Having to eat differently from their peers is not something they'll be thrilled about. Part of your job as a parent may be to make your teens see they're not the only ones having to deal with this disease.

Many online resources are available for kids and teens. We discovered a few really neat websites, and some offer links and other resources for kid-friendly celiac information. Here are a few:

- G-free Kid: gfreekid.com

- KidsHealth: kidshealth.org/kid/nutrition/diets/celiac.html

- Celiac Sprue Association Cel-Kids Network: csaceliacs.info/children.jsp

- Celiac Disease Foundation Support for Teens and Kids: celiac.org (click the Kids tab)

- National Foundation for Celiac Awareness Kids Central: celiaccentral.org/kids (Also check out the series of "Pep Talks" for kids and by kids: celiaccentral.org/kids/pep-talks.)

- Celiac Teen: celiacteen.com (The author started her blog when she was younger, but she still has great posts about teenager-hood and celiac disease.)

Being a supportive parent who understands the difficulty a teen is experiencing can help along the way. Also, keeping the lines of communication open when a teen is experiencing stress about food, friends, and life can go far.

> **FOOD FOR THOUGHT**
>
> The older your child gets, the harder it might be for gluten-free eating all the time. Be prepared for a teen to feel the need to try glutenous foods. Keep providing support and resources as you sense this time coming. As high school graduation nears, other resources, including blogs written by and for college-age students, recommend how to shop and eat gluten free. Research these and other sites to share with your teen.

Most teens tend to disappear to hang out with friends, but still establish time to spend cooking or grocery shopping with your teen. If nothing else, you're helping lay the foundation for a lifelong focus on gluten-free eating.

Gluten-Free Living at College

Colleges and universities are becoming more accommodating for those who need to eat gluten free. In fact, as with picking out a gluten-free camp, when a student is shopping for a university, investigate a school's gluten-free options as much as the residence hall amenities.

Some university students are even starting their own gluten-free student clubs in campus communities. Many college kids are blogging about their gluten-free experiences and providing helpful resources.

The National Foundation for Celiac Awareness devotes a large portion of its website to "Going to College Gluten-Free" and offers *GREAT U: A Gluten-Free Guide to College Living,* an online magazine geared toward college-age celiac sufferers and advice from a parent of two gluten-free college students. Log on to celiaccentral.org/college to learn more.

The Least You Need to Know

- Provide your gluten-intolerant child's school with a copy of the doctor's written prescription for his gluten-free diet.
- Deal with going to a children's birthday party much as you would going to your own friend's dinner party; call the host to RSVP and discuss gluten-free foods.
- Discuss your child's gluten-intolerant diet with school administrators, nurses, teachers, and any and all other caregivers who interact with your child.
- Many fun and educational online resources can help your child understand gluten intolerance.

CHAPTER 12

Thriving on a Gluten-Free Diet

Having to change your diet, cutting out a food or ingredient you've relied on for years, is a big deal. For many of us, meals are some of the most social interactions we enjoy, and often holidays and other parties focus on foods—Fourth of July barbecues, Memorial Day picnics, Thanksgiving dinners, etc.

In this chapter, we help you navigate these changes as you educate your family and friends about your gluten-free lifestyle and the changes you're making.

Many websites, forums, and in-real-life communities can help you manage these changes, too. In fact, you might find a few new friends who share your food intolerances and with whom you can start building your own buddy system and small support group.

One of the best ways to thrive without gluten is to master your kitchen and take charge of your own cooking. Preparing your own gluten-free meals means you can expand your options and puts you in control over your health. And that's really what this is all about.

In This Chapter

- Dealing with change
- Embracing your new diet and lifestyle
- Gluten-free cooking
- Tempering cravings

Feeling in Charge

When you're told you must give up something, obviously you need time to adjust to the change. Being newly diagnosed as gluten intolerant, you need to figure out how to move forward while leaving behind wheat, barley, or rye—which might have been mainstays in your daily meals. Remember, having a diagnosed issue with gluten requires you never to eat gluten again—ever.

Part of feeling in charge is to surround yourself with people who support your goal of letting go of gluten. Keep those folks who don't want to understand what you're up against on the sidelines until you can feel you have control over your new lifestyle change.

Getting Support

Hopefully, when you were diagnosed, your medical practitioner gave you a list of resources to help you get started eating gluten free. If not, request a referral from your doctor for the name of a dietitian who can guide you through your transition.

A dietitian can connect you with local support groups or websites to give you information. She may even give you a recommendation for a meal plan, which can put you on the right path. Our meal plan in Chapter 8 can help extend the meal plan she provides.

Health food stores and cooperatives often provide or facilitate classes about various health issues, including gluten-free eating. Ask at the customer service desk if anything is scheduled. These folks might also be able to put you in touch with someone who tests gluten-free samples for them. That person might also be able to make product recommendations for you, as well as give you ideas about the local gluten-free community.

For Elizabeth, one awesome local resource for learning about gluten-free eating and meeting other people is a community food education resource center. Ryanna Battiste is a community educator, and her business, Grub (thisisgrub.com), provides classes, workshops, and consultations that help change people's relationships with food. In addition, Grub hosts monthly gatherings and classes by local educators, and an on-staff culinary nutritionist leads fun cooking classes.

Battiste explains, "Something so simple as learning how to pan sear a steak [and] make a quick and delicious sauce is so empowering as we learn to shake off the 'rules' in the kitchen and start having fun with our food."

Grub also hosts food-free challenges. One challenge is to live 3 weeks without sugar or nearly 2 months eating only healthy, whole food. The beauty of these challenges is they challenge you as an individual while providing you the support of a group and connection within the community. Battiste explains, "Research shows that having support and accountability, even in the form of a signed agreement with yourself that is shared in confidence with a small group sets you up for success in making those changes."

FOOD FOR THOUGHT

When making a change, encouragement and accountability—even if shared with a small group of people—sets you up for success.

You might want to work with a consultant or health coach, too. A gluten-free health coach can help you plan grocery shopping and accompany you to the grocery store to help you find healthy, whole foods. Some consultants even help you clear your pantry of glutenous goods.

As you explore these different areas of help and support, you'll soon discover that gluten-free food becomes the common theme and something to share together. By reaching out for support, you'll start building your own network of gluten-free friends.

Explaining the Changes to Friends

Maybe you've had digestive issues all your life. Perhaps you've had health issues caused by your gluten intolerance. Whatever your situation, changing your diet might be the one element you can identify that can change your life, your outlook, and your health.

When you make such a big change, your body will show it. Elizabeth felt better when she shifted from gluten to gluten free. A friend of hers, whose medical practitioner suggested she also remove gluten, lost 20 pounds when she made the change. She also feels better and attributes her improved health to relinquishing gluten.

As a parent, sometimes your child is the reason you're exploring gluten-free eating, and while it helps her feel better, it also makes the rest of the family feel better, too. Battiste's experiences with gluten started with her son's extreme colic. Medical professionals told her she should stop breastfeeding because her son was "allergic" to her breast-milk. After doing some research and talking to other moms, she learned a mother's diet can trigger a child's colic. So she started removing food from her diet to help her son. At the same time, she started feeling profoundly better, and lifelong physical and mental symptoms slipped away. She then received a diagnosis of celiac.

"Even though I was good with food and cooking, I underwent an extreme metamorphosis while sorting out what I was able to enjoy for the rest of my life, who was going to be supportive, and what relationships needed to be let go, and grieving the loss of soft springy sweet call of gluten," Battiste says now. Connecting to others helped lift Battiste out of the self-pity she experienced after her diagnosis, and now her passion toward helping others has led to her thriving health and business.

The point is, outside of sharing meals, your friends and family will notice the changes in you and that extra spring in your gluten-free step. When they comment on this, nicely and politely offer to educate them, too, and remain open to their questions. Your new lifestyle might just inspire them to take steps to solve a health problem they have.

TASTY TIDBIT

Ensure that your friends and family understand how they can help you stick with gluten-free eating. If you clearly explain your needs, they'll be more likely to help you succeed. But emphasize you'd like their *help,* not their *hovering.*

Sometimes when Elizabeth has explained she doesn't eat gluten, a friend might try to overprotect her. Be clear about what you need. Often Elizabeth doesn't need protection but rather understanding that her not eating someone's fruitcake isn't a rejection of that friend or their food. She's simply avoiding gluten.

Even though you'll be creating new friendships with other gluten-intolerant people, keep your regular support group strong by sharing with them how your lifestyle and eating habits have changed and how they can support you. One way to encourage that is to share some of your gluten-free food with them. In Chapter 10, we give you tips on entertaining gluten free. When you invite guests, make a point of explaining how exciting this change is in your life and how pleased you are to share it with them. Infectious enthusiasm is hard to beat!

Through your support group or dietitian, if you've made friends with other gluten-intolerant people, invite one or two. This way, you can start integrating your long-term support group with your new group of supportive, gluten-free friends.

A New Mind-Set

Going gluten free is like trying on a new set of clothes. Even if, in reality, you're keeping your old clothes, you'll soon see how much better your body feels in the new ones.

When you feel better, your mind-set will shift. One of Elizabeth's symptoms was brain fog. Not eating gluten helped her improve her focus, which gave her another benefit to ridding gluten from her diet.

GLUTEN GAFFE

If you aren't feeling better, you might need to talk with your doctor or dietitian. Also keep a close eye on what you're eating to see if you're accidentally eating hidden gluten.

Finding a Food Community

After a couple years of being gluten free, Elizabeth found her food community. They exist as a mixture of local people she interacts with:

- On Facebook

- At health food stores or gluten-free bakeries

- At her children's school

- At cooking classes

- Standing behind someone at the grocery checkout ("Excuse me, is that a good gluten-free chocolate-chip cookie?")

- At friends' parties

- At community events focused on healthy living

- At gluten-free Meetup groups

Elizabeth also has a nonlocal community she interacts with on Twitter, various blogs (see Appendix B for suggestions), and community forums. Look around, and you'll find gluten-free communities you can be part of as well.

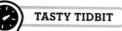 **TASTY TIDBIT**

Ask at your local health food store, or search social media for local gluten-free events to start building your own gluten-free community. One place to check for events in your area is the Gluten-Free Calendar (glutenfreecalendar.com).

Elizabeth created her food community by just reaching out, asking questions, and finding answers to her questions. To get a conversation started, she might ask, "Where can I find fresh baked gluten-free bread?"

Battiste explains, "Making those 'practical application' changes is really hard when first coming off gluten. Finding bread that doesn't taste like cardboard and learning how to cook a meal instead of ripping open a box and microwaving it can be seriously daunting. At Grub, we have found that those who tap into the community, ask questions, share recipes, and throw themselves into the information, scary as it is, have a much easier time than their isolated counterparts."

One key component Battiste has seen time and time again is that even though people know they need to make a change, they won't change until they're ready. She's also seen proof that people change faster and are more assured when they have a community who supports them.

Finding a Food Buddy

Do you need a food buddy to go gluten free? No, not necessarily. But Elizabeth transformed her supportive husband into her food buddy after he experienced gluten-free eating and then had tests to confirm he also reacts to gluten.

A gluten-free food buddy is not a requirement. But having one can be a big help. You're eating gluten free for life. Having someone's support helps increase your chances for success. Also, you get to encourage and share your knowledge with someone as well.

For example, maybe your buddy likes a certain brand of fish sticks. You've just read an article about gluten-free and learned the fish stick manufacturer is changing its recipe to include barley flakes. By sharing that information, you ensure your friend is aware of the change. Or maybe you learn a local restaurant is opening and offering gluten-free options. Sounds like the perfect opportunity for you and your friend to make a date to visit the new restaurant.

One of the ways Elizabeth has capitalized on a food buddy is sharing gluten-free food. Ordering a large bag of gluten-free flour is cheaper by the pound, so she'll buy a large amount and split the flour and cost with her buddy. This also can encourage swapping recipes, and discussing what's on your friend's menu can lead to trying different gluten-free options.

Battiste mentions, "Like any massive life shift and change, having support is critical to a successful outcome. Taking out gluten is no easy feat for many reasons. Because it is so addicting, that initial shift away can produce some serious anxiety and cravings."

Knowing you have someone you can talk to about a topic that's often an isolating experience can make a big difference. In Battiste's experience, her clients' own food issues became authentic when they met others with the same issues. These encounters helped create and sustain motivation for those involved. And this can be the case in online meetings, too.

Battiste says, "This is the community, the online community, which has truly helped millions understand the impact of food on their health. As more people blogged, chatted, posted recipes, and commented on posts, we have forged a massive web of sharing and empowerment."

Joining a National Organization

Many national awareness and support organizations have local branches. To find one near you, check with these organizations:

- Celiac.com—search for "celiac support groups"

- Celiac Disease Foundation and chapters (celiac.org)—look under Support

- Celiac Sprue Association (csaceliacs.info)—look under Get Involved for local chapters

- Canadian Celiac Association (celiac.ca)—look under The CCA for local chapter lists
- Gluten Intolerance Group (www.gluten.net/local-branches)

If you don't find a chapter or group in your area, consider starting one and create your community through helping others to learn about gluten intolerance.

FOOD FOR THOUGHT

Approximately 1 in 133 people suffers from celiac disease, which means someone in your city or immediate community also eats gluten free.

Embracing Gluten-Free Cooking

We spend a lot of time—too much time—focused on quick-and-easy dinners. Unfortunately, you may have to slow your meal preparations as you cook gluten-free meals because you'll be relying less on packaged foods and more on fresh, whole foods.

Make use of the 90+ recipes we share in Part 4, and also spend time researching and finding other cookbooks for your taste, budget, and know-how. Remember, living gluten free will become easier!

Coping with Changing Your Diet

As you shift your diet and start feeling better, you might think if you cheat, it won't hurt you. But with gluten, a little bit *can* hurt. If you can remember this, you'll have an easier time letting go of gluten. Is a doughnut *that* important to you? Is it worth it knowing you'll get sick? Or can you eat some filling almonds and raisins instead? Having this conversation with yourself can help you make the gluten-free decision.

In the first few weeks, you'll be frustrated and wish you'd never heard of gluten. Rely on your network of friends to help you through. Let them know if and when you're having difficulty coping. When people care about you, they want you to be happy and healthy. Rely on that, and let folks know what you need.

When going gluten free, making time to plan meals helped Elizabeth the most. She had to figure out what she could cook that was relatively easy and quick, so she made gluten-free pasta during a busy part of the week and a roast chicken with hearty sides when she knew she'd have more time.

Your planning includes shopping for healthy, gluten-free, whole foods and filling the pantry with ingredients you can use. When you've spent the money and have the foods handy, you're less likely to alter your plans and splurge on dinner out where you might cheat or be glutened.

Eating with Family—Without Making Two Meals

When eating with your family, you might think two separate meals would be the best option. Or maybe you think you'll buy the prepackaged foods for your family but eat your own freshly prepared meal. Remember, your health considerations may also impact your family—celiac disease is genetic. So make one simple meal everyone can eat.

Battiste concurs, "We all need something a bit different, but there is one common thread to what we need: REAL FOODS. Food as nature intends us to eat."

With so many couples and families working out of the home these days, our lives are busy. Elizabeth has a friend who, because of busy schedules, feeds each child dinner at a different time every night. However, the mother makes only one meal, which she serves from 4 P.M. onward.

If your schedule doesn't allow for cooking dinner at night because of scheduling demands, investigate slow cookers. Keep fresh vegetables available to serve on the side. Or cook in bulk to eat throughout the week and defrost along the way. "There is nothing a healthy dose of creativity, positive attitude, and community support cannot fix," Battiste says.

Dealing with Food Cravings

If you haven't already, you'll soon learn one gluten-free day might be better than the next. Becoming gluten free means you'll be eating different foods and trying some new foods you never thought would pass your lips.

Expect to experience cravings. They're part of this transition you're making. One way to approach a craving is to just let it pass and start working on something else for a little while. (Most food cravings pass within 20 minutes.) The craving should diminish as you focus on something else.

 TASTY TIDBIT

Food cravings will happen. Have a plan for when they do—find a gluten-free substitute, replace with another treat, or focus on something else until the craving is gone.

Also, look at your cravings as an opportunity and a challenge to find gluten-free replacements for the glutenous comfort foods you used to enjoy. As you cook and prepare a variety of foods, you'll soon notice you miss your previous glutenous foods less and less.

Not sure where to start? Check your local library for gluten-free or Paleo cookbooks. Or borrow a book from a gluten-free friend. You also could search the internet for "gluten-free" and the food you want to replace, such as "bread" or "lasagna." Find some recipes and try them out. Start simple, and as your knowledge and confidence increases, add to your repertoire. As you try more and more new gluten-free foods, you'll crave glutenous items less often.

Elizabeth is still trying to find a gluten-free licorice, but she substitutes with another treat. For example, she easily replaced an annual treat—a glutenous tiramisu recipe and any cravings along with it—by preparing the recipe printed on the gluten-free Schär Ladyfingers package.

Does your family love your lasagna? Experiment with different gluten-free lasagna noodles—packaged or homemade—and have them tell you what they like best about each one.

The Least You Need to Know

- Part of feeling in charge is to surround yourself with people who support your goal of gluten-free eating.
- Find gluten-free communities around you—a mixture of local and online folks you can interact with.
- One way to deal with cravings is to find a gluten-free recipe for the food you crave.

Gluten-Free Recipes

In Part 4, you put everything you've learned so far into action with all the healthy gluten-free recipes we've included.

We start with some of the basics, giving you a reason to smile as you wake up for a healthy breakfast. We also dress up some terrific lunchtime salads with a colorful array of ingredients and give you several delicious dressing recipes. When you need a snack, you'll love the gluten-free options we give you. And for dinner, elegant, hearty dinner recipes round out your day.

Even though you're kicking gluten to the curb, you don't have to say so long to pasta and bread. We've provided several crowd-pleasing recipes, even for those still eating gluten.

And who said anything about giving up dessert because of gluten? In the final chapter, we give you several delectable desserts to put the finishing touch on your gluten-free menu.

One final note: if you're eating a specific diet in addition to going gluten free, we've included icons with the recipes that appeal to kids, are vegan-friendly, and fit within the guidelines of the Paleo diet. There's something for everyone!

CHAPTER 13

Good-Morning Breakfasts

Now that you've got the basics of gluten-free eating down pat, it's time to get cooking, and there's no better place to begin than breakfast.

Pancakes, crepes, cereal, and more—the good-for-you breakfasts in this chapter get you up and going. We also include some suggestions for making your morning meals easier to prepare (because who has extra time on hurried weekday mornings?). In addition, we include some easy substitutions you can make if you or your loved ones have other food sensitivities.

In This Chapter

- Tips for making breakfast easy
- Simple substitutions
- Grab-and-go morning meals

Breakfast Basics

Breakfast is the most important meal of the day. You've probably heard that before, but it's true. Your body needs something nourishing to break the fast of the past 8 or so hours you were asleep, and you need something healthy to fuel you through your morning until lunch. Unfortunately, gluten is a common ingredient in many mainstream breakfast dishes, so you've got to think outside the box a bit when it comes to your morning meal.

You could start with some protein-rich eggs. They cook quickly for busy mornings, and they'll keep you going until your midday meal. For quick-and-easy mornings, cook some eggs the night before and tuck them in the freezer for portable breakfast the next morning. Serving sizes of scrambled eggs and small omelets freeze well for quick reheating. Poached and fried eggs don't come through the freezing-and-thawing process well.

If you're a cereal person, stock up on gluten-free cereals, including creamy hot rice cereals, oatmeal, and granolas. Gluten-free breads are great for toast, and you can find gluten-free bagels in some specialty stores. Use them to make your own egg sandwiches—perfect to make ahead, freeze, and grab on your way out the door to work or school.

Most toaster pastries and frozen breakfast wraps are gluten minefields. Instead, shop for gluten-free versions in specialty stores—or avoid them completely. If you're a big pancake or waffle fan, double or triple the recipes later in this chapter, and freeze individual portions to enjoy when you don't have time to prepare them from scratch.

Two common breakfast food ingredients you might be a bit unfamiliar with are *quinoa* and *buckwheat*. Quinoa is a grainlike seed, that also comes in flake form, which looks like oatmeal and tastes like nutty, hearty oatmeal. You can substitute quinoa flakes for gluten-free oatmeal if you're especially sensitive, and they're also good added to baked goods. Buckwheat, despite the name, isn't actually wheat but a plant related to rhubarb. It offers a nutty, hearty taste that's perfect for breakfast dishes, especially pancakes and waffles.

> **DEFINITION**
>
> **Quinoa** is a gluten-free seed used like rice or barley and also comes in flake form, similar to oatmeal. **Buckwheat,** a gluten-free seed that can be ground into flour, offers a hearty, whole-grain taste. Both are good any time of day but especially at breakfast.

What about frozen breakfast potatoes? They should be fine, right? Not necessarily. Some contain just potatoes or potatoes and salt, but others contain glutenous starches, so read the labels. If you like hash browns, peel some fresh potatoes, chop them in a food processor, and freeze them in breakfast-size portions to fry as you want them.

Most breakfast meats like sausage, bacon, and ham are made completely from gluten-free ingredients—meats, spices, and preservatives. But some are made in facilities that also process gluten-filled products. In general, buy meats that have simple labels with real foods. Jeanette likes Trader Joe's chicken sausages because they don't contain preservatives or nitrates and other additives. Elizabeth's family enjoys Pederson's Natural Farm bacons and sausages. About.com's celiac disease page, celiacdisease.about.com, offers an updated list of many popular gluten-free brands. Or talk with your local butcher about his meats; he can tell you where he got the meat, what he added, and how they've been handled every step of the way.

If you don't have any nut allergies, try LÄRABARs for a grab-and-go meal. They fit perfectly into purses and glove compartments, and are one of your best bets for breakfasts on the go.

Breakfast Substitutions

We use eggs in several of our recipes, but if you have an allergy, consider using a mixture of 3 tablespoons water with 1 tablespoon flaxseed meal. It's a simple replacement used in many vegan recipes. Your pancakes and waffles will have more fiber and be a bit healthier, too. (Check Chapter 3 for more egg substitutions.) If you want to make an egglike casserole without eggs, scramble some herbed tofu with vegetables and sausage, and top it with vegan cheese.

Several recipes use butter. If you avoid butter, you can replace it with coconut oil or a vegan margarine.

Replace milk with hemp, soy, almond, rice, or coconut milk. Jeanette uses coconut and almond milk because they're rich and delicious, even the unsweetened, plain versions. Elizabeth's family uses hemp and almond milk as dairy replacements.

Our Grain-Free Peanut Butter Granola recipe contains peanut butter. If you have a peanut allergy, you can replace the peanut butter with almond or other nut butters.

And you can make any of our recipes with no spices or more spices, no salt or more salt, and no sugar or more sugar. Or you can replace sugar with honey, maple syrup, and agave syrup. But take note—all three substitutions tend to taste sweeter than straight sugar, so start with half an amount and add more to taste.

✪ ✪ Cinnamon Maple Quinoa Cereal

This sweet and creamy cereal offers a little cinnamony kick to get your day started right. It's also a great replacement for those glutenous instant oatmeal packages. But best of all, it's just as easy to prepare.

Yield:	Prep time:	Cook time:	Serving size:
1 cup	1 minute	1 minute	1 cup

Each serving has:				
260 calories	2.5g fat	2.5g saturated fat	0mg cholesterol	79mg sodium
28g sugar	49g carbohydrates	2.4g fiber	4.3g protein	

$^1/_3$ cup dry quinoa flakes	2 TB. maple syrup
$^1/_2$ cup water	$^1/_2$ tsp. cinnamon
$^1/_2$ cup plus 3 TB. coconut milk	$^1/_2$ tsp. vanilla extract

1. In a deep, microwave-safe bowl, combine quinoa flakes, water, and $^1/_2$ cup coconut milk. Microwave on high for 1 minute.

2. Stir quinoa flakes, and mix in remaining 3 tablespoons coconut milk, maple syrup, cinnamon, and vanilla extract. Enjoy.

Variation: You can add 1 tablespoon dried almonds for crunch, swap out the cinnamon for $^1/_2$ teaspoon nutmeg, substitute brown sugar or honey for the maple syrup. And you don't need to use coconut milk—you can cook the quinoa flakes all in water, or you can use regular milk or another kind of milk.

 TASTY TIDBIT

If you're quite busy, you can make individual proportions of this cereal and simplify the recipe. In small zipper-lock plastic bags, combine $^1/_3$ cup quinoa flakes, $^1/_2$ teaspoon cinnamon, and 1 tablespoon brown sugar. Toss in your briefcase or purse, and at the office, pour the mixture into a bowl, add the milk or water, and microwave. Instant breakfast!

✪ Sausage, Cheese, and Spinach Breakfast Casserole

Savory and filling, this casserole is a great addition to special brunches and weekend breakfasts.

Yield:	Prep time:	Cook time:	Serving size:
1 (9-inch-square) casserole	15 minutes	45 to 50 minutes	$^1/_4$ casserole

Each serving has:				
376 calories	25g fat	9.5g saturated fat	68mg cholesterol	483mg sodium
3g sugar	18g carbohydrates	2g fiber	17g protein	

4 slices gluten-free bread

$^1/_2$ lb. bulk pork breakfast sausage

1 small onion, sliced

$^1/_2$ tsp. extra-virgin olive oil (optional)

5 large eggs

1 cup frozen spinach, thawed and squeezed

$^1/_4$ cup nonfat milk

$^1/_2$ cup grated cheddar cheese or crumbled chèvre

Sea salt

Freshly ground black pepper

1. Preheat the oven to 350°F.

2. Place slices of gluten-free bread in a 9-inch-square cake pan. Set aside.

3. In a large cast-iron or nonstick skillet over high heat, sauté sausage for about 5 to 8 minutes or until cooked. Remove sausage from the skillet using a slotted spoon, leaving drippings in the skillet.

4. Reduce heat to medium-high, add onion and extra-virgin olive oil (if drippings aren't enough). Sauté for about 5 minutes or until just browned. Remove from heat.

5. In a food processor fitted with a standard S-blade, pulse eggs, spinach, milk, and $^1/_4$ cup cheddar cheese for about 2 minutes or until spinach is chopped and eggs, milk, and cheese are well mixed. Add cooked onion, and pulse for 1 or 2 minutes or until finely chopped and combined.

6. Crumble sausage, stir into egg mixture, and season with sea salt and black pepper. Pour over bread slices, and sprinkle with remaining $^1/_4$ cup cheddar cheese.

7. Bake for 25 to 30 minutes or until puffed and golden on top, like a soufflé.

Variation: Instead of sausage, you can use bacon, ham, or even cooked chicken. You can also add cooked broccoli, mushrooms, or red peppers.

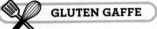 **GLUTEN GAFFE**

Because both cheese and sausage contain salt, you might not want to add any additional salt.

❽ Buckwheat Buttermilk Pancakes with Strawberry Balsamic Syrup

Hearty yet fluffy, these pancakes (or waffles) are so good, you'll want to make a double batch so you can freeze the extras for later. The homemade strawberry syrup is sweet with just a bit of tang to wake it up.

Yield:	Prep time:	Cook time:	Serving size:
16 pancakes or 4 waffles, 1^1/$_2$ cups syrup	15 minutes	45 minutes	4 pancakes or 1 waffle plus 2 tablespoons syrup

Each serving has:

361 calories	8.7g fat	5g saturated fat	21mg cholesterol	327mg sodium
15g sugar	61g carbohydrates	6g fiber	13g protein	

2^1/$_2$ cups low-fat buttermilk	^{1}/$_2$ cup white rice flour
2 large eggs	2 tsp. baking powder
2 TB. unsalted butter or coconut oil, melted	^{1}/$_2$ tsp. baking soda
2 TB. maple syrup	^{1}/$_4$ tsp. xanthan gum
2 tsp. vanilla extract	1 tsp. cinnamon
1^1/$_2$ cups buckwheat flour	1 batch Strawberry Balsamic Syrup (recipe later in this chapter)

1. Preheat a griddle or waffle maker to high.

2. In a large bowl, whisk together buttermilk, eggs, melted butter, maple syrup, and vanilla extract.

3. In another large bowl, stir together buckwheat flour, white rice flour, baking powder, baking soda, xanthan gum, and cinnamon.

4. Gradually whisk dry ingredients into wet ingredients until well combined.

5. When griddle or waffle maker is hot, brush with a little melted butter or spray with cooking spray. Pour ^{1}/$_2$ to ^{3}/$_4$ cup batter onto griddle or waffle maker (depending on the size of your waffle maker), and cook for about 4 or 5 minutes or until done.

6. Remove cooked pancake or waffle to a plate, keep warm, and continue on with remaining batter. Serve with Strawberry Balsamic Syrup.

TASTY TIDBIT

Instead of low-fat buttermilk, you can use almond milk or coconut milk mixed with 2^1/$_2$ tablespoons vinegar or lemon juice.

✪ Cornmeal Pancakes

This delicious breakfast pleaser tastes similar to cornbread in pancake form. The difference is subtle, but we think you'll like it.

Yield:	Prep time:	Cook time:	Serving size:
12 (3-inch) pancakes	10 minutes	20 minutes	3 pancakes

Each serving has:				
341 calories	9g fat	5g saturated fat	58mg cholesterol	247mg sodium
3g sugar	58g carbohydrates	2g fiber	8g protein	

1 large egg

2 TB. unsalted butter or coconut oil, melted

1^1/$_4$ cups low-fat buttermilk, or 1^1/$_4$ cups nondairy milk plus 1 TB. vinegar or lemon juice

1 tsp. vanilla extract

1^1/$_3$ cups gluten-free flour blend

^{1}/$_2$ cup cornmeal

1 TB. sugar

2 tsp. baking powder

^{1}/$_2$ tsp. baking soda

^{1}/$_4$ tsp. xanthan gum

1. Preheat an electric griddle to 400°F. Spray with cooking spray or brush with a little melted butter.

2. In a large bowl, whisk together egg, melted butter, buttermilk, and vanilla extract.

3. In another large bowl, stir together gluten-free flour blend, cornmeal, sugar, baking powder, baking soda, and xanthan gum.

4. Gradually, stir dry ingredients into wet ingredients until well combined.

5. Pour batter onto the griddle by the ^{1}/$_4$ cup. Cook for about 2 or 3 minutes or until tiny bubbles begin to form on top of pancake. Flip over pancake, and cook for 2 more minutes. Serve with maple syrup.

 TASTY TIDBIT

To prepare these pancakes faster, use an electric mixer to combine all ingredients. Still mix the wet ingredients and the dry ingredients separately before combining them.

⊗ Gluten-Free Crepes with Caramelized Bananas

Delicate yet spongy, these crepes will transport you to on the banks of the Seine. They're especially delicious topped or filled with the simple caramelized banana recipe featured in this recipe.

Yield:	Prep time:	Cook time:	Serving size:
12 crepes	20 minutes	45 minutes	3 crepes

Each serving has:				
450 calories	22g fat	12g saturated fat	127mg cholesterol	231mg sodium
15g sugar	56g carbohydrates	5g fiber	11g protein	

^{2}/$_3$ cup buckwheat flour

^{1}/$_3$ cup white rice flour

2 TB. tapioca starch

1 TB. white sugar

^{1}/$_4$ tsp. sea salt

^{1}/$_4$ tsp. xanthan gum

1^1/$_2$ cups 2 percent milk

2 eggs

4 TB. plus 4 TB. clarified butter, melted

6 large bananas, peeled and sliced into ^{1}/$_2$-in. slices

1. In a large bowl, whisk together buckwheat flour, white rice flour, tapioca starch, white sugar, sea salt, and xanthan gum.

2. Whisk in 2 percent milk, eggs, and 4 tablespoons clarified butter until no clumps remain. If mixture seems especially clumpy, add 1 or 2 extra tablespoons milk. You want a batter that's smooth and not too thick.

3. Heat a small crepe pan or 8-inch nonstick skillet over high heat for 1 minute. Brush with a little clarified butter. Pour ^{1}/$_4$ cup batter onto the pan, and rotate the pan so a batter covers the pan in a thin layer. Cook for about 2 minutes or until bubbles start to form on crepe. Using a spatula, flip over crepe, and cook for 1 more minute. Slide onto plate, brush pan with clarified butter, and repeat with remaining batter.

4. Heat a large, nonstick or cast-iron pan over high heat for at least 2 minutes. When pan is hot, add 1 or 2 tablespoons clarified butter to the pan, and add bananas in a single layer. You might have to do this in batches.

5. Fry bananas for 2 or 3 minutes on one side until golden brown. Using a spatula, flip over bananas, and cook for 2 more minutes. Carefully remove from the pan. Repeat with remaining bananas, adding a little more clarified butter, if needed.

6. To serve, place about 2 or 3 tablespoons caramelized bananas in the middle of 1 crepe, and fold over. Top with whipped cream or maple syrup, if desired.

Variation: You can serve these crepes with savory ingredients, too, like chicken and mushrooms sautéed in wine. Simply omit the 1 tablespoon sugar from the recipe.

TASTY TIDBIT

Clarifying butter removes the water and milk solids, making it better for sautéing foods like crepes. If you use whole butter, the milk solids will burn, which isn't what you want when making crepes. To clarify, cut $1^1/_2$ sticks butter into cubes, and melt in a small saucepan over medium-high heat. Let the butter simmer, and do not stir. After the water evaporates, you'll see bubbling clouds of milk solids. Remove from heat, and pour the melted butter through a fine-mesh strainer lined with a damp cheesecloth. The solids will stay on the cloth, and the clarified butter will slip right through. This might seem like a lot of work, but it's so worth it.

⊕ ⊗ Great Granola

This crunchy, sweet granola is packed with dried fruits, nuts, and seeds. Serve it alone with milk, or mix it with yogurt and fruit.

Yield:	Prep time:	Cook time:	Serving size:	
10 cups	20 minutes	45 minutes	$^1/_2$ cup	
Each serving has:				
214 calories	10.9g fat	2g saturated fat	0mg cholesterol	22mg sodium
11g sugar	26.4g carbohydrates	3.6g fiber	4.2g protein	

$3^1/_2$ cups gluten-free oats

$1^1/_2$ cups gluten-free rice cereal

$^1/_2$ cup chopped almonds

$^1/_2$ cup chopped pecans

$^1/_2$ cup chopped hazelnuts

$^1/_4$ cup pumpkin seeds

$^1/_4$ cup sunflower seeds

$^1/_8$ cup flaxseeds

$^1/_8$ cup sesame seeds

$^1/_2$ cup dried cranberries

$^1/_2$ cup dried apricots, chopped

$^1/_2$ cup dried cherries

$^3/_4$ cup shredded coconut

Zest from 2 medium oranges (4 TB.)

1 TB. fresh squeezed orange juice

$^1/_2$ cup brown sugar, firmly packed

$^1/_3$ cup molasses

$^1/_3$ cup maple syrup

$^1/_4$ cup grapeseed oil

1 tsp. vanilla extract

2 tsp. cinnamon

1 tsp. nutmeg

1. Preheat the oven to 350°F.

2. In a very large bowl, combine oats, rice cereal, almonds, pecans, hazelnuts, pumpkin seeds, sunflower seeds, flaxseeds, sesame seeds, cranberries, apricots, cherries, coconut and 2 tablespoons orange zest.

3. In a large saucepan over medium-high heat, bring remaining 2 tablespoons orange zest, orange juice, brown sugar, molasses, maple syrup, grapeseed oil, vanilla extract, cinnamon and nutmeg to a boil, stirring until mixture boils. Remove from heat.

4. Pour syrup mixture over seed mixture, and stir until well combined.

5. Spread granola in an even layer on several baking sheet sheets (about 4). Bake for 45 minutes, stirring every 10 minutes. Watch the edges because they tend to get done faster; after 25 to 30 minutes, you might want to scrape them into a bowl. Granola is done when lightly brown and crisp.

6. Cool to room temperature, and store in an airtight container for up to 1 month.

 TASTY TIDBIT

Granola became popular in the 1970s, but it actually was a food for invalids back in the late 1800s. This version is adapted from Napa Valley, California's Inn on Randolph.

✪ Grain-Free Peanut Butter Granola

Thanks to the peanut butter, coconut, honey, and vanilla, this granola is so flavorful and addictive, you'll find it hard not to lick the bowl.

Yield:	Prep time:	Cook time:	Serving size:
6¹/2 to 7 cups	2 minutes	15 to 20 minutes	1 cup

Each serving has:				
260 calories	9g fat	2.6g saturated fat	0mg cholesterol	7mg sodium
21g sugar	38g carbohydrates	8.5g fiber	7g protein	

2 cups gluten-free rolled oats or flaked quinoa

¹/2 cup ground flaxseeds

¹/2 cup dried coconut flakes

¹/4 cup sunflower seeds

¹/2 cup unsweetened peanut butter

¹/2 cup honey

1 TB. vanilla extract

1. Preheat the oven to 350°F.

2. In a large bowl, combine gluten-free rolled oats, flaxseeds, coconut flakes, and sunflower seeds.

3. Stir in peanut butter, honey, and vanilla extract until well combined. Spread in an even layer on 2 baking sheets.

4. Bake for 15 to 20 minutes, stirring every 5 minutes, or until granola is dark golden in color. Remove from the oven, and let cool for 10 minutes.

5. Store in zipper-lock plastic bags at room temperature for up to 1 month.

Variation: You can substitute almond butter for the peanut butter. You can add 1 teaspoon cinnamon if you like.

 TASTY TIDBIT

You can make this recipe in a food dehydrator. Instead of spreading the mixture on baking sheets, spread it on the dehydrator trays. Dry at 145°F for 8 to 14 hours. The resulting granola will have intensified peanut and vanilla flavors.

❂ ✪ Strawberry Balsamic Syrup

Sweet and summery with just a touch of tang from the vinegar, this syrup makes an outstanding topper for pancakes, waffles, and French toast. It's equally great atop chicken breasts, too.

Yield:	Prep time:	Cook time:	Serving size:
1¹/₂ cups	10 minutes	20 minutes	2 tablespoons

Each serving has:				
15 calories	0g fat	0g saturated fat	0mg cholesterol	1mg sodium
2g sugar	4g carbohydrates	1g fiber	0.2g protein	

1 (1-lb.) bag frozen, unsweetened strawberries, thawed	2 tsp. vanilla extract
1 TB. pure maple syrup	2 tsp. balsamic vinegar
	¹/₂ tsp. cinnamon

1. In a food processor fitted with a standard S-blade, purée about 1 cup strawberries for about 2 minutes.

2. In a medium saucepan over medium-high heat, heat puréed strawberries and remaining whole strawberries, stirring frequently, for about 5 minutes.

3. When thickened and reduced, add maple syrup, vanilla extract, balsamic vinegar, and cinnamon, and cook, stirring frequently, for 3 or 4 more minutes.

Variation: You can omit the balsamic vinegar if you like. Instead of cinnamon, you can use nutmeg. And for fun, drop in a few chocolate chips.

 TASTY TIDBIT

For a gourmet touch, add 2 tablespoons chopped, fresh basil or mint. Basil goes especially well with strawberries and balsamic vinegar.

CHAPTER 14

Sensational Salads and Dressings

Sure, it's easy enough to grab a bag of mixed greens as you walk through the grocery store's produce section, but wait. Some bagged salads contain gluten-enhanced toppings. Well, finding a bottle of dressing should be simple, right? Not so. Many prepared dressings contain gluten-laden thickeners and additives.

You don't have those problems with homemade salads and salad dressings. When you make your own, you customize the ingredients and use only what you know for sure is gluten free. Plus, they're easy and fun to make.

In this chapter, we teach you the basics of building great salads and share easy ways to whip up fresh dressings, too. We even show you how to add fancy touches for special occasions.

In This Chapter

- Assembling super salads
- Making mouthwatering dressing
- Advanced salad-making ideas

Building a Better Salad

Lettuce, the main ingredient in most salads, comes in many varieties. Iceberg is nice and crisp, but it's also kind of boring, so if you want your salads to spring with flavor, try romaine, red leaf, arugula, and baby spinach. Or try mixing baby spinach with Boston or romaine with red leaf. This contrast of color and texture is a very simple way to spruce up your salads.

Bright orange carrots, vibrant red bell peppers, and glowing yellow squashes add a splash of color and good-for-you nutrition. Choose whatever veggies are fresh and in season, and add tomatoes when they're ripest at the end of summer.

For one serving of a basic mixed green salad, blend 1 or 2 cups lettuce and $^1/_2$ to 1 cup chopped veggies. Buy organic and local veggies whenever possible because they taste best.

 TASTY TIDBIT

Rinse whatever produce you choose thoroughly with water before adding to your salad. To avoid waterlogging lettuce and veggies, use a salad spinner, or shake them out in a colander and dry lightly with paper towels.

Salads aren't only for veggies. You also can add fruits—dried, fresh, or even canned—for a pop of sweetness and color. Dried cherries and cranberries, fresh apples and pears, or canned mandarin oranges are flavorful additions. Jeanette likes a salad made of mixed greens, kalamata olives, mandarin oranges, cherry tomatoes, fresh balls of mozzarella, and Paul Newman's Italian dressing. (It's gluten-free!) Jeanette later re-created the salad using her own Italian dressing.

Dressing Up Your Salad

Making homemade salad dressing isn't difficult. In fact, salad dressings are some of the easiest condiments you'll ever make. They're basically just an emulsion of oil and vinegar with flavorings added.

The easiest vinaigrette is 3 parts oil to 1 part vinegar (try $^3/_4$ cup oil to $^1/_4$ cup vinegar) with either sea or kosher salt added along with black pepper. This recipe is for an entire salad, but if you're just making a lunch for yourself, you can easily store this salad dressing in a covered container for up to a week in the refrigerator.

That 3-to-1 ratio isn't set in stone, however. Jeanette prefers less oil—a 1-to-1 ratio—especially because the calories in oil wallop those in vinegar. If you're counting calories, reduce the amount of oil, but do it to your taste. And if you're concerned about calories but don't like too much vinegar, start with a 1-to-1 ratio of vinegar to oil. Add more oil gradually, by the tablespoon, to see what you prefer.

As you reduce the amount of oil, you need to add another liquid to make up for the vinegar. You could add water, for example, or try fruit juices, which add another level of flavor and complexity.

Because the dressing base has only two components, choose good-quality oil and vinegar. Extra-virgin olive oil is perfect for salad dressings, but a more neutral or basic vegetable oil works well, too. Walnut and other nut oils add a nutty depth to dressings, and grapeseed oil is a nice, neutral oil as well. When it comes to vinegar, opt for a cider or balsamic vinegar, which are sweeter and have more flavor. White or red wine vinegars, sherry vinegar, and raspberry vinegar can be fun, too. When you start making your own dressings, try different vinegars and oils and see what suits your taste.

For seasoning, use sea salt or kosher salt. Regular table salt, while salty, doesn't add as much flavor. You can use preground black pepper, but using a pepper grinder adds a more flavorful punch of flavor.

If your dressing recipe includes dried herbs and spices, check them before using to see if they contain anticaking agents, which have gluten. The Spice House (thespicehouse.com) is one very good source for almost entirely gluten-free spices (only two items it sells contains gluten). Its garlic and onion powders are certifiably gluten free, and its vanillas, smoke powders, salad dressing bases, and spice blends are as well. Penzeys (penzeys.com) is another good spice company that does not add or process gluten in its spices or herb blends. Its soup bases, however, do contain gluten.

 TASTY TIDBIT

Spices generally don't last more than a year. Before using, sniff a spice to see if it's old. If it gives off only a faint aroma, toss it. Old spices add nothing to your dressings or sauces.

Some dressings call for fresh garlic or shallots, and many call for Dijon mustard—a fabulous condiment that's almost always gluten free. Both The Spice House and Penzeys sell dried, minced shallots, a great salad dressing enhancer. It's worth having on hand if you make dressings and sauces from scratch.

Finally, some dressings call for a sweetener. Sugar, honey, and maple syrup add sweetness to a vinaigrette. If a vinaigrette tastes too tart, adding a teaspoon or two of sugar can sweeten it without overpowering it.

Getting Fancy

Once you master the basics of making salads and dressings, you can get fancy. For example, consider adding cooked vegetables. Roasted squashes, caramelized onions, and sautéed mushrooms add a lot of *oomph* to a salad. Jeanette recently enjoyed a salad of cooked portobello mushrooms on mixed greens with just a touch of goat cheese and truffle oil drizzled on top.

You can also cook fruits for your salads. Poached apples and pears taste sublime over mixed greens with a simple vinaigrette.

Or think about adding cheeses, meats, or fish. Fresh goat cheese, crumbled cheddar cheese, and even little bits of Brie can add a bite of savory flavor and a softer texture. Choose a good cheese, and add no more than an ounce or two for an entire salad. A little bit goes a long way.

 FOOD FOR THOUGHT

> When dressing up your salads, think about the foods and flavors you love. If you adore salmon and pistachios, add them with a honey mustard or basic vinaigrette. If you love steak, add it to a Caesar salad. Go with your favorite tastes, and have fun experimenting.

When it comes to meat, try adding special hams, crumbled bacon, and grilled chicken breasts. If you have steak left over from dinner, toss it into your salad for a complete meal. Or add bacon to your lunch salad. The same goes for that leftover salmon. It tastes great with greens.

Why not add something crunchy, too? Nuts, cashews, pecans, pistachios, hazelnuts, and almonds all taste great in salads. Sunflower seeds and pumpkin seeds also add a nice crunch. Adding nuts and dried fruits elevate your salad from average to spectacular.

☻ Crunchy Asian Quinoa Salad

This salad sings with sweetness, color, and crunch. It's bursting with antioxidant-rich vegetables, and the quinoa packs quite a protein punch. Sweet and crunchy with just a touch of gingery tang, this salad is quite addictive!

Yield:	Prep time:	Cook time:	Serving size:
10 cups	45 minutes, plus 1 hour marinate time	30 minutes	1 cup salad, 1 cup greens, 1 tablespoon almonds, plus 1 tablespoon zesty sprouts

Each serving has:

248 calories	9g fat	1g saturated fat	0mg cholesterol	245mg sodium
14g sugar	37g carbohydrates	6g fiber	7g protein	

$1^1/_2$ cups water

1 cup red quinoa

4 to 6 large napa cabbage leaves, diced (3 cups)

1 large red bell pepper, ribs and seeds removed, and diced (2 cups chopped)

1 medium cucumber, diced (2 cups)

1 large carrot, peeled and grated (about $1^1/_2$ cups)

4 oz. pea pods, diced (1 cup)

1 bunch green onions (about 8), green parts only, diced (1 cup)

$^1/_4$ cup fresh cilantro, minced

4 seedless mandarin oranges, peeled and segmented, or 1 (11-oz.) can mandarin oranges, drained

1 TB. orange zest

$^1/_2$ cup rice vinegar

$^1/_4$ cup toasted sesame oil

$^1/_4$ cup unsweetened applesauce

$^1/_4$ cup honey

3 cloves garlic, minced

1 (3-in.) piece fresh ginger, peeled and grated (1 TB.)

2 TB. tamari soy sauce

2 tsp. Dijon mustard

Freshly ground black pepper

Pinch cayenne

10 cups mixed greens

$^1/_2$ plus 2 TB. toasted, slivered almonds

$^1/_2$ plus 2 TB. spicy sprouts or *microgreens*

1. In a medium saucepan over high heat, bring water to a boil. Add red quinoa, stir, cover, and reduce heat to medium-low. Simmer for about 30 minutes or until quinoa is soft and water is absorbed. (If you have a rice cooker, you can cook quinoa as you would cook rice.)

2. Meanwhile, in a large bowl, combine napa cabbage, red bell pepper, cucumber, carrot, pea pods, green onions, cilantro, and mandarin oranges.

3. In a medium bowl, whisk together orange zest, rice vinegar, toasted sesame oil, applesauce, honey, garlic, ginger, tamari soy sauce, Dijon mustard, black pepper, and cayenne. Set aside.

4. Pour cooked quinoa into a large bowl, and let cool for at least 10 to 15 minutes. When quinoa is no longer steaming, mix it into chopped vegetables. Pour dressing over top, and stir to combine. Refrigerate for 1 hour to let flavors meld.

5. To serve, place 1 cup mixed greens in each bowl. Top with 1 cup vegetable-quinoa mixture, 1 tablespoon almonds, and 1 tablespoon spicy sprouts.

Variation: If you can't find toasted sesame oil, regular sesame oil works just as well. You can also substitute with extra-virgin olive oil in a pinch. Toasting your own almonds is easy: heat a medium pan over high heat for 2 minutes, add slivered almonds, and cook, stirring every 20 seconds to prevent burning, for about 2 to 4 minutes or until almonds become golden in color and smell toasted.

DEFINITION

Microgreens are tiny, edible vegetables and herbs harvested when they're only 1 to 1$^1/_2$ inches long with tiny green leaves. Long prized by chefs, they pack a wallop of a flavor for their size. You can find these at some larger supermarkets and also at health food stores.

❂ ❂ Roasted Asparagus Salad

This is a delicious, springy salad that features the savory, roasted asparagus.

Yield:	Prep time:	Cook time:	Serving size:
10 cups	45 minutes, plus 1 hour marinate time	15 minutes	1 cup salad, 1 cup greens, 1 table-spoon almonds, plus 1 tablespoon zesty sprouts

Each serving has:				
70 calories	4g fat	0.5g saturated fat	0mg cholesterol	160mg sodium
4g sugar	7g carbohydrates	3g fiber	2g protein	

¼ large red onion, sliced sliver-thin

1 large bunch asparagus stalks, ends removed (about 24 stalks)

1 TB. extra-virgin olive oil

1 TB. balsamic vinegar

Sea salt

Freshly ground black pepper

1 medium head red or green leaf lettuce, shredded

1 large red bell pepper, ribs and seeds removed, and sliced thin

1. Place red onion slivers in a small bowl of water, and set aside to soak for 15 minutes.

2. Meanwhile, preheat the oven to 350°F.

3. Arrange asparagus stalks on a baking sheet. Drizzle with extra-virgin olive oil and balsamic vinegar, and sprinkle with sea salt and black pepper. Bake for 15 minutes.

4. To assemble salad, place 2 cups lettuce in each bowl. Divide red bell peppers evenly among bowls.

5. Drain onion slivers, and divide evenly among bowls.

6. Place 6 stalks asparagus on each salad, and serve with your choice of dressing. Balsamic vinaigrette works well with this salad.

Variation: For extra crunch, add some chopped almonds or pecans to the salad, and for extra sweetness, add some dried cranberries or cherries—about 1 tablespoon each per bowl.

 TASTY TIDBIT

Roasted asparagus doesn't just taste good in salads. It's also a great side for dinners, and it's good chopped and added to sandwiches and wraps as well.

☉ ☻ Simple Kale Salad

Sweet and almost herbal with just a touch of salt, this is one of my family's absolute favorites.

Yield:	**Prep time:**	**Serving size:**		
4 cups	2 minutes	1 cup		
Each serving has:				
103 calories	7.5g fat	1g saturated fat	0mg cholesterol	176mg sodium
2g sugar	8g carbohydrates	2g fiber	2g protein	

2 large bunches Tuscan kale	2 tsp. sugar
2 TB. balsamic vinegar	$^1/_4$ tsp. sea salt
2 TB. walnut oil	$^1/_4$ tsp. freshly ground black pepper

1. Using clean hands, pull Tuscan kale leaves from stalks. Discard stalks. Tear kale leaves into bite-size pieces, and place in a large bowl.

2. Pour balsamic vinegar and walnut oil over kale leaves, and massage with your fingers.

3. Add sugar, sea salt, and black pepper, massage again.

4. Divide evenly among 4 bowls, and serve.

 TASTY TIDBIT

Tuscan kale, also known as lacinto kale, is the kale that comes in big, dark green leaves. You can substitute with curly kale or Swiss chard, too. Although it sounds strange, massaging the oil, vinegar, salt, sugar, and pepper into the kale leaves tenderizes the leaves and really gives this salad its flavor and texture.

☻ Caesar Salad

Peppery yet creamy, savory yet tangy, this classic salad is wonderful as an entrée all by itself, especially if you add meat or fish.

Yield:	Prep time:	Cook time:	Serving size:
8 cups	15 minutes	1 minute	2 cups

Each serving has:				
233 calories	22g fat	3g saturated fat	41mg cholesterol	123mg sodium
3g sugar	9g carbohydrates	2g fiber	3g protein	

1 large egg	$^1/_8$ tsp. sea salt
$^1/_4$ cup extra-virgin olive oil	1 large head romaine lettuce, outer leaves removed, inner leaves washed and chopped (about 8 cups)
Juice of 1 large lemon (3 TB.)	
2 cloves garlic, crushed	
2 tsp. Dijon mustard	$^1/_3$ cup Parmegiano Reggiano or Grana Padano cheese, grated
$1^1/_2$ tsp. anchovy paste	
1 tsp. capers	1 batch Homemade Croutons (recipe later in this chapter)
1 tsp. Worcestershire sauce	
$^1/_2$ tsp. freshly ground black pepper	

1. Fill a small saucepan with water, and bring to a boil over medium-high heat. Gently place egg into water, and boil for 1 minute. Remove the saucepan from heat.

2. In a food processor fitted with a standard S-chopping blade, add extra-virgin olive oil, lemon juice, garlic cloves, Dijon mustard, anchovy paste, capers, Worcestershire sauce, black pepper, and sea salt.

3. Crack coddled egg into the food processor, scraping even the white cooked bits from the shell. Pulse for 1 or 2 minutes or until everything is combined.

4. To assemble salad, toss romaine lettuce, dressing, Parmegiano Reggiano cheese, and Homemade Croutons in a large bowl, and serve immediately.

Variation: For more than just a simple Caesar salad, toss in mushrooms, kalamata olives, red onions, red bell peppers, and cherry tomatoes. Use whatever amounts you like, from $^1/_2$ to 1 cup veggies.

 GLUTEN GAFFE

The egg used in this recipe is only coddled (only cooked a little, and not hard-boiled), so be sure to use eggs from a source you trust. Pasteurized eggs are one option. Cage-free eggs are also good because the hens are less likely to be contaminated.

Balsamic Vinaigrette

Slightly sweet and tart, this dressing is perfect for a simple salad of mixed greens. It's also good with tomatoes, fresh basil, and fresh mozzarella.

Yield:		Prep time:	Serving size:	
²/₃ cup (10 ¹/₂ tablespoons)		2 minutes	2 tablespoons	
Each serving has:				
125 calories	14g fat	2g saturated fat	0mg cholesterol	59mg sodium
28g sugar	0.6g carbohydrates	0g fiber	0g protein	

¹/₃ cup extra-virgin olive oil

¹/₃ cup balsamic vinegar

1 TB. fresh shallots, minced, or 1 TB. dried

2 tsp. honey

2 tsp. Dijon mustard

¹/₄ tsp. freshly ground black pepper

¹/₈ tsp. sea salt

1. In a medium bowl, whisk together extra-virgin olive oil, balsamic vinegar, shallots, honey, Dijon mustard, black pepper, and sea salt.

2. Toss or drizzle over salad or refrigerate for up to 1 week.

Variation: The 1:1 ratio of oil to vinegar might be too tart for some. If you think it tastes too tart, add more oil, 1 tablespoon at a time, until it reaches the taste you prefer. You can also add 1 or 2 tablespoons cherry or cranberry juice to lessen the tartness.

 FOOD FOR THOUGHT

Balsamic vinegar is good for salads. You also can toss it with cooked green beans. It's also tasty added to carrots, parsnips, rutabagas, and other root vegetables before you cook them. You even can use it to flavor chicken breasts and fish.

⊗ Ranch Dressing

This tangy, creamy dressing isn't just for salads. It's great with a wide variety of other foods, too.

Yield:	Prep time:	Serving size:
1 cup (16 tablespoons)	5 minutes	2 tablespoons

Each serving has:				
56 calories	3g fat	0g saturated fat	3mg cholesterol	70mg sodium
5g sugar	6g carbohydrates	0g fiber	1g protein	

½ cup low-fat buttermilk

¼ cup gluten-free mayonnaise

3 TB. apple cider vinegar

2 TB. extra-virgin olive oil

2 TB. sugar

1 TB. Dijon mustard

1 tsp. dried parsley

1 tsp. onion powder

1 tsp. garlic powder

¼ tsp. celery seed

¼ tsp. dried dill

Sea salt

Freshly ground black pepper

1. In a medium bowl, whisk together buttermilk, mayonnaise, apple cider vinegar, extra-virgin olive oil, sugar, Dijon mustard, parsley, onion powder, garlic powder, celery seed, dried dill, sea salt, and black pepper.

2. Toss or drizzle over salad or refrigerate for up to 1 week.

Variation: For **Southwestern Ranch Dressing,** add 2 tablespoons fresh salsa and 1 tablespoon fresh cilantro and process in a food processor fitted with a standard S-blade for 2 minutes.

 TASTY TIDBIT

This dressing is great as a sandwich spread, and it's also a good dip for cut veggies, chips, and especially for homemade french fries.

✿ ☻ French Dressing

This sweet and tart dressing not only adds zing to your salads, but it can also be used as a dip or sauce for chicken breasts and baked fish.

Yield:		Prep time:	Serving size:	
²/₃ cup (10 tablespoons)		5 minutes	2 tablespoons	
Each serving has:				
180 calories	21g fat	1.6g saturated fat	0mg cholesterol	20mg sodium
0g sugar	0.1g carbohydrates	0g fiber	0g protein	

¹/₂ cup grapeseed, canola, or other neutral-tasting oil

¹/₄ cup apple cider vinegar

2 TB. sugar

1 tsp. dry mustard powder

1 tsp. smoked paprika

1 tsp. garlic powder

¹/₂ tsp. onion powder

¹/₂ tsp. celery seeds

Sea salt

Freshly ground black pepper

1. In a medium bowl, whisk together grapeseed oil, apple cider vinegar, sugar, dry mustard powder, smoked paprika, garlic powder, onion powder, celery seeds, sea salt, black pepper.

2. Toss or drizzle over salad. Or refrigerate for up to 1 week.

Variation: For **Catalina-Style French Dressing,** add 1 tablespoon tomato paste, 1 additional tablespoon sugar, and 2 additional tablespoons apple cider vinegar. For a **Creamy Poppy Seed French Dressing,** add ¹/₂ to 1 teaspoon poppy seeds.

 TASTY TIDBIT

This is a great dressing to serve over iceberg lettuce wedges with sprinklings of freshly cooked bacon and blue cheese. Just be sure the blue cheese is gluten free.

☻ Honey Mustard Dressing

Sweet with honey and tangy with mustard, this dressing adds a zip to your salads.

Yield:	Prep time:	Serving size:
¹/₂ cup (8 tablespoons)	5 minutes	2 tablespoons

Each serving has:				
156 calories	13g fat	1.8g saturated fat	0mg cholesterol	75mg sodium
9g sugar	10g carbohydrates	0g fiber	0.7g protein	

¹/₄ cup extra-virgin olive oil	1 tsp. onion powder
¹/₄ cup apple cider vinegar	¹/₂ tsp. garlic powder
2 TB. honey	Sea salt
1 TB. Dijon mustard	Freshly ground black pepper

1. In a medium bowl, whisk together extra-virgin olive oil, apple cider vinegar, honey, Dijon mustard, onion powder, garlic powder, sea salt, and black pepper.

2. Toss or drizzle over salad. Or refrigerate for up to 1 week.

 TASTY TIDBIT

Honey mustard is a tasty dip for chips and a super spread for sandwiches. It's also fabulous tossed over chicken breasts or salmon fillets before you bake them.

✪ Blue Cheese Dressing

Tangy and tart, this blue cheese dressing is terrific served over mixed greens. It's also a great dip for chicken wings. And best of all, it's pretty low calorie for a blue cheese dressing!

Yield:	Prep time:	Serving size:		
³/₄ cup	5 minutes	2 tablespoons		
Each serving has:				
66 calories	5.3g fat	2.2g saturated fat	8mg cholesterol	183mg sodium
1.2g sugar	1.8g carbohydrates	0g fiber	2.9g protein	

2 oz. blue cheese

¹/₂ cup low-fat buttermilk

1 TB. extra-virgin olive oil

1 TB. apple cider vinegar

1 TB. Dijon mustard

¹/₂ tsp. onion powder

¹/₂ tsp. garlic powder

¹/₂ tsp. fresh ground black pepper

1. In a food processor fitted with a standard S-blade, process blue cheese, low-fat buttermilk, extra-virgin olive oil, apple cider vinegar, Dijon mustard, onion powder, garlic powder, and black pepper for 1 or 2 minutes or until well blended.

2. Toss with salad.

Variation: If you really love blue cheese, after blending this dressing, stir in 2 more ounces blue cheese diced small. For an herbal edge, add 1 tablespoon minced fresh chives and 1 tablespoon minced fresh parsley.

TASTY TIDBIT

This dressing is a perfect partner for the classic wedge salad. To make a wedge salad, cut 1 head iceberg lettuce into 4 wedges. Top with chopped roma or cherry tomatoes (about ¹/₄ cup per salad) and chopped bacon (about 2 tablespoons bacon per salad), and additional blue cheese chunks (about 2 ounces per salad).

◉ Asian Ginger Dressing

This sweet and gingery dressing adds an exotic touch to simple greens.

Yield:	Prep time:	Serving size:		
$^2/_3$ cup	5 minutes	2 tablespoons		
Each serving has:				
108 calories	8.6g fat	1.3g saturated fat	0mg cholesterol	153mg sodium
6.5g sugar	8g carbohydrates	0g fiber	0.4g protein	

$^1/_4$ cup sesame oil	1 TB. tamari
3 TB. rice vinegar	2 cloves garlic
2 TB. lemon juice	1 ($1^1/_2$-in.) piece fresh ginger, peeled
2 TB. sugar	

1. In a food processor fitted with a standard blade, process sesame oil, rice vinegar, lemon juice, sugar, tamari, garlic, and ginger for 2 minutes or until smooth.

2. Toss or drizzle over salad. Or refrigerate for up to 1 week.

Variation: For an extra tang of flavor, add 1 teaspoon tomato paste.

 TASTY TIDBIT

A great basic salad for this dressing is 6 to 8 cups mixed greens, $^1/_2$ cup chopped pea pods, $^1/_2$ cup chopped cucumbers, and $^1/_2$ cup grated carrots. Top with toasted sesames or toasted almonds.

Homemade Croutons

These garlicky croutons taste great in the Caesar salad, but they brighten up almost every other kind of salad, too.

Yield:	Prep time:	Cook time:	Serving size:
2¹/₂ cups croutons	5 minutes	15 minutes	¹/₂ cup

Each serving has:				
112 calories	7.5g fat	1g saturated fat	0mg cholesterol	94mg sodium
0g sugar	10g carbohydrates	1g fiber	0g protein	

4 slices gluten-free bread, toasted and cut into 1¹/₂-in. cubes (about 2¹/₂ cups)

2 TB. extra-virgin olive oil

1 tsp. onion powder

1 tsp. garlic powder

¹/₄ tsp. sea salt

¹/₄ tsp. Cajun seasoning

1. Preheat the oven to 350°F.

2. In a large bowl, gently toss bread cubes, extra-virgin olive oil, onion powder, garlic powder, sea salt, and Cajun seasoning.

3. Spread croutons in a single layer onto a cookie sheet. Bake for 15 minutes, stirring at least once, until golden brown in color.

4. Remove from the oven, and toss into salad. Or store in an airtight container at room temperature for up to 2 weeks.

 TASTY TIDBIT

Although this recipe was made to go with the Caesar salad recipe, these croutons can top any salad. They're equally fantastic dunked in soup, especially French onion soup topped with cheese.

CHAPTER 15

Sassy Snacks and Sauces

Most potato chips and some sauces are gluten free, but many familiar snacks are unfortunately now out of reach on a gluten-free diet. But never fear. You still can satisfy your cravings and make your own—without gluten. Not only are you able to snack and sauce things up as your taste buds dictate, but your snacks and sauces will be fresher and more delicious because you made them.

In this chapter, we give you some quick and easy snack and sauce recipes you and your family will love.

In This Chapter

- Super snacks
- Nutritional noshes
- Sensational sauces

✴ ⓥ Almond and Sesame Energy Bars

This sweet, slightly salty, crunchy, nutty bar is so delicious it's hard to eat just one. It's a great treat to have on hand to grab when you're on the go.

Yield:	Prep time:	Cook time:	Serving size:	
10 bars	15 minutes	20 minutes	1 bar	

Each serving has:				
320 calories	23g fat	2.6g saturated fat	0mg cholesterol	52mg sodium
14g sugar	24g carbohydrates	5g fiber	9g protein	

$^1/_2$ cup almonds	$^1/_2$ cup honey
$^1/_2$ cup unsweetened dried coconut	3 TB. ground flaxseeds
$1^1/_2$ cups sesame seeds	1 tsp. vanilla extract
$^1/_2$ cup sunflower seeds	$^1/_4$ tsp. sea salt
$^1/_2$ cup almond butter	

1. Preheat the oven to 325°F. Line a $9^1/_2 \times 9^1/_2$-inch baking pan with parchment paper.

2. In a food processor fitted with a standard S-blade, pulse together almonds and dried coconut for about 4 or 5 minutes or until you have a nice, crumbly mixture.

3. In a large bowl, stir together sesame seeds, sunflower seeds, almond butter, honey, and flaxseeds. Add almond-coconut mixture, and stir in vanilla extract and sea salt.

4. Press bar mixture into the prepared pan. Bake for 20 minutes. Remove from the oven, and cool on the counter for 20 minutes.

5. Cover the pan, and refrigerate for at least 1 hour. Remove from the refrigerator, and slice into bars. Store in an airtight container.

Variation: You also can add $^1/_2$ cup dried cranberries with the sesame seeds.

 TASTY TIDBIT

This bar was inspired by the expensive energy bars Jeanette used to buy at her coop. They're easy to make, and they freeze well in individual portions so you have to-go snacks whenever you need them.

⊕ ❁ Homemade Popcorn with Truffle Oil

The heady aroma of truffles adds a savory note to this quick and easy snack.

Yield:	Prep time:	Cook time:	Serving size:	
6 cups	1 or 2 minutes	10 minutes	2 cups	

Each serving has:				
58 calories	6g fat	0.6g saturated fat	0mg cholesterol	156mg sodium
2g sugar	24g carbohydrates	4g fiber	4g protein	

1 TB. canola oil	1 tsp. truffle oil
⅔ cup popcorn kernels	Sea salt

1. In a medium lidded pan over medium-high heat, heat canola oil. Add 4 test popcorn kernels, cover, and wait 1 or 2 minutes for test kernels to pop.

2. After kernels pop, remove the pot from heat, add remaining popcorn kernels, cover, shake the pot to distribute kernels evenly, and return the pot to the stove. Pop kernels, shaking the pot every minute. When there are 2 or 3 seconds between pops, remove the pot from heat.

3. Pour popcorn into a large bowl, drizzle with truffle oil, season with sea salt, and enjoy.

Variation: You can add 2 tablespoons grated Parmesan cheese for an extra boost of flavor.

 FOOD FOR THOUGHT

Many truffle oils aren't made from actual truffles—they are made from chemicals. For the real stuff, check out oregontruffleoil.com.

⦿ ⦿ Kale Chips

This crunchy snack packs a powerful vitamin punch, along with a bit of spice.

Yield:	Prep time:	Cook time:	Serving size:	
3 or 4 cups	10 minutes	15 minutes	$1^1/_2$ to 2 cups	
Each serving has:				
127 calories	7g fat	1g saturated fat	0mg cholesterol	1,120mg sodium
3g sugar	9g carbohydrates	2.7g fiber	4.4g protein	

1 large bunch Tuscan kale, stems removed, leaves torn into large pieces	1 tsp. sea salt
	1 tsp. Cajun seasoning
1 TB. extra-virgin olive oil	

1. Preheat the oven to 350°F.

2. In a large bowl, combine Tuscan kale leaves, extra-virgin olive oil, sea salt, and Cajun seasoning. Spread leaves over large, nonstick baking sheet.

3. Bake for 15 minutes, remove from the oven, cool for 5 minutes, and serve.

Variation: Instead of Cajun seasoning, you can use garlic powder, onion powder, or whatever other spices you like.

 TASTY TIDBIT

Kale is a powerhouse green. It's packed with antioxidants, vitamin C, vitamin K, vitamin A, and lots of fiber.

⊕ ⊗ Healthy Hummus

This garlic- and lemon-laced chickpea dip is delicious with anything from crackers to veggies.

Yield:	Prep time:	Serving size:		
2 cups	10 minutes	3 tablespoons		
Each serving has:				
238 calories	13g fat	2g saturated fat	0mg cholesterol	21mg sodium
4g sugar	25g carbohydrates	7g fiber	9g protein	

2 cups chickpeas, drained and
  rinsed if canned

4 cloves garlic

¹/₂ cup tahini

¹/₄ cup extra-virgin olive oil

3 TB. fresh squeezed lemon juice

1. In a food processor fitted with a standard S-blade, purée chickpeas, garlic, tahini, extra-virgin olive oil, and lemon juice for 2 or 3 minutes or until puréed.

2. Serve with crackers, bread cubes, or fresh vegetables.

Variation: For **Roasted Red Pepper Hummus,** add 2 or 3 roasted red peppers and ¹/₈ teaspoon Spanish sweet paprika to the food processor.

TASTY TIDBIT

Most canned chickpeas contain salt, so you might want to skip adding any extra sodium. If the finished hummus doesn't taste right to you, season with just a little sea or kosher salt.

❁ Ginger Carrot Dip

This tangy dip is sweetened by orange juice and honey in addition to the carrots. It tastes great spread on crackers, bread, and crudités.

Yield:	Prep time:	Cook time:	Serving size:
3 cups	30 minutes, plus 1 hour marinate time	2 hours	¼ cup

Each serving has:				
155 calories	1g fat	0g saturated fat	0mg cholesterol	345mg sodium
7g sugar	31g carbohydrates	3g fiber	4g protein	

6 to 8 medium carrots, peeled and diced (4 cups)

3 cloves garlic, minced

2 TB. sherry wine vinegar

2 TB. honey

2 TB. fresh squeezed orange juice

2 TB. fresh grated ginger

Zest of 1 medium orange (about 1 TB.)

Pinch cayenne

Sea salt

Fresh ground pepper

1 TB. fresh parsley, finely minced

1. Bring large pot of water to a boil over medium-high heat. Drop in carrots, and boil for about 15 minutes or until tender. Drain and rinse with cold water.

2. In a large bowl, whisk together garlic, sherry wine vinegar, honey, orange juice, ginger, orange zest, and cayenne. Add carrots, cover, and refrigerate for 1 hour to marinate.

3. In a blender or a food processor fitted with a standard S-blade, puree carrots and marinade for 5 minutes.

4. Season with sea salt and black pepper, sprinkle with parsley, and serve.

Variation: If you don't have sherry wine vinegar, you can use the same amount of apple cider vinegar instead.

 TASTY TIDBIT

This dip makes delightful canapés. Spoon 1 teaspoon Ginger Carrot Dip on top of a slice of cucumber and set on a small round of gluten-free bread. Sprinkle with a few parsley leaves, and enjoy. You can also top radish slices the same way.

ⓦ ❸ Walnut Tofu Pate

This savory, garlicky, and oniony dip is great for veggies and crackers, but you can also spread it on sandwiches in place of hummus or mayo.

Yield: 2³/₄ cups	Prep time: 2 minutes	Cook time: 30 minutes	Serving size: 1 tablespoon	
Each serving has:				
20 calories	1.5g fat	2.6g saturated fat	0mg cholesterol	32mg sodium
0g sugar	0.9g carbohydrates	less than 1g fiber	1.3g protein	

16 oz. firm tofu

¹/₃ cup walnuts

¹/₃ cup cashews

4 tsp. tamari

3 tsp. onion powder

2 tsp. garlic powder

1 tsp. dried thyme

1 tsp. fresh lemon juice

1. In a food processor fitted with a standard S-blade, purée tofu, walnuts, cashews, tamari, onion powder, garlic powder, thyme, and lemon juice for 5 minutes.

2. Place pate in a bowl, cover, and refrigerate for at least 1 hour to let flavors meld. Serve with your favorite gluten-free crackers, or spread on sandwiches.

 TASTY TIDBIT

Before you use the tofu, first drain it from the water it's stored in. Then gently press the tofu with a paper towel to squeeze out excess water. If you don't get rid of the water, the spices won't flavor the tofu as strongly.

✪ Basic Mayonnaise

This creamy, slightly lemony mayo is so delicious you may never buy the jarred stuff again.

Yield:	Prep time:	Serving size:		
2 cups	20 minutes	1 tablespoon		

Each serving has:				
141 calories	16g fat	2g saturated fat	20mg cholesterol	22mg sodium
12g sugar	0.1g carbohydrates	0g fiber	0.3g protein	

3 egg yolks

$2^1/_2$ cups extra-virgin olive oil or
    canola oil

1 TB. freshly squeezed lemon juice

1 TB. Dijon mustard

Sea salt

Freshly ground white pepper

1. In a medium bowl, whisk egg yolks for about 2 or 3 minutes or until light.

2. Add a tiny drizzle of extra-virgin olive oil—less than $^1/_2$ teaspoon—and whisk briskly for 1 or 2 minutes or until well blended. Add another drizzle of olive oil, and whisk again until well blended. Keep drizzling and whisking very, very slowly so yolks and olive oil emulsify.

3. After oil and yolks have all been incorporated into a paste, add lemon juice, Dijon mustard, sea salt, and white pepper, and mix well. Use immediately or refrigerate.

Variation: To make **Garlic Aioli Sauce,** whisk in 2 or 3 cloves minced garlic with the lemon juice. For **Lemon Mayonnaise,** add the juice and zest of $^1/_2$ lemon. Both sauces are great for topping vegetables, poultry, and seafood.

FOOD FOR THOUGHT

It might not seem like you're making much progress as you drizzle in a tiny amount of oil and whisk it into the yolks, but as you do this, the oil and yolks will gradually thicken and become the consistency of the spreadable mayo you find in jars. If you have any concerns about food safety regarding the use of raw egg yolks, use pasteurized eggs.

ⓦ ✪ Homemade Ketchup

Sweet, tangy tomato goodness with a depth of spice, homemade ketchup tastes so much better than anything you get from a bottle. This recipe comes from Jeanette's friend Chef Jeff King.

Yield:	Prep time:	Cook time:	Serving size:	
about 2$\frac{1}{2}$ cups	15 minutes	1 hour, 45 minutes	1 tablespoon	
Each serving has:				
19 calories	1g fat	0g saturated fat	0mg cholesterol	91mg sodium
2.8g sugar	3.1g carbohydrates	0g fiber	0.1g protein	

1 (28-oz.) can whole tomatoes in purée	$\frac{1}{2}$ cup cider vinegar
2 TB. water	1 tsp. garlic powder
2 TB. extra-virgin olive oil	$\frac{1}{4}$ tsp. allspice
1 medium onion, chopped	$\frac{1}{4}$ tsp. cloves
1 TB. tomato paste	1 tsp. sea salt
$\frac{3}{4}$ cup dark brown sugar, firmly packed	

1. In a blender, purée tomatoes, including purée sauce, until smooth. Add water if necessary to reach a smooth consistency.

2. In a 4-quart heavy saucepan over medium heat, heat extra-virgin olive oil. Add onion, and cook, stirring often, for about 8 minutes or until softened.

3. Add puréed tomatoes, tomato paste, dark brown sugar, cider vinegar, garlic powder, allspice, cloves, and sea salt. Reduce heat to low, and simmer, stirring occasionally, for about 1 hour or until very thick.

4. Remove from heat and allow to cool for 15 to 20 minutes.

5. Pour $\frac{1}{2}$ of ketchup into a blender, and blend until smooth. Transfer to a storage container, and repeat with remaining ketchup.

6. Cover and chill for at least 2 hours before serving. Ketchup will keep for several days in the refrigerator.

Variation: For a **Spicy Ketchup,** add $^1/_2$ teaspoon cayenne. For **Umami Ketchup,** add a few drops truffle oil to 1 cup Homemade Ketchup. For **Cocktail Sauce,** add 1 dash Worcestershire sauce, 1 teaspoon horseradish sauce, and 1 teaspoon fresh squeezed lemon juice to 2 tablespoons Homemade Ketchup.

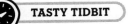

TASTY TIDBIT

The average North American eats more than 65 pounds of ketchup every year.

☻ Best Barbecue Sauce

This easy-to-make barbecue sauce tastes tangy, sweet, and just slightly smoky.

Yield:	Prep time:	Cook time:	Serving size:
2 cups	2 minutes	20 minutes	2 tablespoons

Each serving has:				
52 calories	0.1g fat	0g saturated fat	0mg cholesterol	94mg sodium
11g sugar	13g carbohydrates	0.6g fiber	0.6g protein	

1 (6-oz.) can tomato paste	1 TB. onion powder
1 cup water	1 TB. ground mustard powder
$^{1}/_{2}$ cup apple cider vinegar	2 tsp. garlic powder
$^{3}/_{4}$ cup packed brown sugar	2 tsp. smoked Spanish paprika
3 TB. molasses	1 tsp. ground cinnamon
2 TB. Worcestershire sauce	$^{1}/_{2}$ tsp. sea salt
1 TB. liquid smoke	Pinch chili powder

1. In a medium saucepan over medium heat, whisk together tomato paste, water, apple cider vinegar, brown sugar, molasses, Worcestershire sauce, liquid smoke, onion powder, mustard powder, garlic powder, Spanish paprika, cinnamon, sea salt, and chili powder. Cook, stirring constantly, for about 15 to 20 minutes. Remove from heat.

2. Use immediately, refrigerate for up to 2 weeks, or freeze for up to 6 months. Serve over roasted meats, grilled meats, and grilled veggies.

Variation: For **Barbecue Ranch Dressing,** mix in an equal amount of homemade Ranch Dressing (recipe in Chapter 14).

 TASTY TIDBIT

Be sure the Worcestershire sauce and liquid smoke you use are gluten free. Call or visit the manufacturer's websites to find out for sure. Lea & Perrins Worcestershire sauce is gluten free, and Colgin's liquid smoke is also gluten free.

Gluten-Free Gravy

Savory, herby, and delicious, this gravy is perfect for Thanksgiving dinner!

Yield:	Prep time:	Cook time:	Serving size:
2 cups	2 minutes	30 minutes	2 tablespoons

Each serving has:				
11 calories	0.1g fat	0g saturated fat	0mg cholesterol	154mg sodium
0g sugar	1.2g carbohydrates	0g fiber	0.1g protein	

2 cups chicken or turkey stock

1 TB. fresh sage, minced

1 TB. fresh thyme, minced

1 TB. fresh savory, minced

1 bay leaf

$^1/_2$ cup white wine

2 TB. cornstarch

Sea salt

Freshly ground white pepper

1. In a medium saucepan over medium-high heat, heat chicken stock, sage, thyme, savory, and bay leaf.

2. In a small bowl, whisk together white wine and cornstarch.

3. Slowly pour cornstarch mixture into chicken stock, and whisk until cornstarch mixture is completely dissolved. Cook, stirring with a wooden spoon, for about 5 to 10 minutes or until thickened and warmed. Season with sea salt and white pepper.

4. Remove bay leaf, and serve.

Variation: Instead of white wine, you can use apple cider, calvados, or regular brandy. If you do not have fresh herbs, use 1 teaspoon each dried herbs.

FOOD FOR THOUGHT

By the time this gravy is finished, it should be the consistency and thickness to coat the back of a spoon.

Béchamel Sauce

This versatile sauce is a great base for creamy soups, and it also can dress up potatoes and vegetables quite nicely. Because you actually infuse the milk with spices, what could be a bland sauce is bursting with savory notes.

Yield:	Prep time:	Cook time:	Serving size:	
2 cups	20 minutes	35 minutes	2 tablespoons	
Each serving has:				
30 calories	2g fat	0g saturated fat	4mg cholesterol	13mg sodium
0g sugar	2g carbohydrates	0g fiber	1g protein	

2 cups 2 percent or whole milk	2 TB. unsalted butter
¼ white onion, peeled but still whole	2 TB. cornstarch dissolved in 2 TB. water
½ tsp. whole cloves	Sea salt
½ tsp. whole peppercorns	Freshly ground white pepper
2 bay leaves	

1. In a medium saucepan over high heat, combine 2 percent milk, white onion, cloves, peppercorns, and bay leaves. Bring to a boil, turn off heat, cover, and infuse for at least 20 minutes.

2. Strain milk through a sieve, discard onion, cloves, peppercorns, and bay leaves.

3. In the same saucepan over medium-high heat, melt butter. Add cornstarch mixture, and stir until combined.

4. Gently whisk in milk, ¼ cup at a time, and cook, stirring, for about 5 to 8 minutes or until sauce thickens. Season with sea salt and white pepper, and serve.

Variation: To make **The Best Cheese Sauce Ever** that's great with vegetables or noodles, add 2 cups grated cheddar, gouda, or your favorite cheese and 2 teaspoons Dijon mustard after the sauce thickens. For an **Even Better Cheese Sauce,** use a mixture of at least two or three different cheeses. Try a blend of fresh chèvre, cheddar, and blue.

 FOOD FOR THOUGHT

The cheese sauces are fantastic for au gratin potatoes and macaroni and cheese. You'll never crave that boxed stuff again.

16

Enticing Entrées and Sides

This chapter focuses on the heart of gluten-free eating—
main courses and side dishes, especially those foods you
think you'll never be able to eat again on a gluten-free diet.
Meatloaf? No longer a problem. Restaurant-style crab cakes?
Not a problem either. And Thanksgiving-worthy stuffing? We
give you not one but two options in this chapter.

In addition, we also share tips on making your own stocks and
take a look at why you should use high-quality ingredients.
The results, as you'll find, are well worth it.

In This Chapter

- Simple strategies for making stocks
- Tips on finding quality ingredients
- Easy ideas for experimenting
- Preparation pointers

Starting with Stocks

The biggest challenge in going gluten-free is that in many cases, you actually have to cook your meals from scratch. So along with selecting the main ingredients, plan to make the sauces and accompaniments to go with them.

Homemade chicken, beef, and vegetable stocks are some of the best ingredients to have on hand when you're cooking—gluten free or otherwise. Stocks were originally designed to use up ripe veggies and meat bones. Once you get the hang of making them, you won't even really need a recipe.

A basic meat stock is just leftover bones and vegetable scraps. Just put the leftover chicken bones, veggies, carrot peels, potato ends, or turnip bits in a pot, and cover with water. Add 1 tablespoon white vinegar, and bring to a boil over medium-high heat. Reduce heat to low, skim off the white and brown icky stuff floating on the top, and cook for 3 to 6 hours. Add a little water as it simmers, and strain out the bones and vegetable bits, and you're done. It's that easy.

FOOD FOR THOUGHT

The vinegar used in making stock draws out the marrow, calcium, and other nutrients from the bones and makes for a richer stock.

Remember to simmer stock—not boil it—for most of the process. As it simmers, impurities work their way to the top where you can strain them off and out of the stock.

The easiest, most basic chicken stock Jeanette makes contains a chicken carcass, 2 or 3 carrots, 1 or 2 onions, 2 leeks, 1 to 3 stalks celery, fresh parsley, fresh thyme, 2 bay leaves, 1 teaspoon black peppercorns, and 1 tablespoon white vinegar. If she doesn't have leeks, she'll substitute turnips. If she doesn't have carrots, she'll add sweet potatoes. Sometimes she'll add spinach or kale or veggie peels. She doesn't worry about doing a perfect dice or chop but just breaks the celery into pieces. If she has no meat bones, she makes a vegetable stock.

The point is, you don't need a perfect ratio or recipe. Whatever you make from scratch will be more delicious than anything you can get from a package.

Opt for Quality

Vegetables grown organically or locally typically taste better than those trucked in from across the globe. And fruits picked at the peak of their season taste sweeter and better not covered in sugar or gluten-filled sauces.

The same holds true for meat and seafood. Shop for these items at butcher shops and specialty stores where you know you'll get the best quality.

High quality should also extend to your spices and herbs. If they're fresh, they'll add taste to your dishes and not detract from them.

Go for Variety

Besides buying good quality, experiment with variety, too. For example, try long-grain rice, short-grain rice, black rice, or wild rice (which actually isn't rice at all). Mix basmati and jasmine, or substitute with arborio. Or substitute quinoa for rice.

Cook with red, green, and yellow lentils. Try black beans, red beans, or pinto beans. Mix them up, and taste them in different quantities together.

By experimenting and broadening your palate, you might discover some new favorites. You'll certainly become more adventurous in your eating.

Healthy Cooking Tips

It's good to keep in mind that just because something is gluten-free doesn't mean it's necessarily healthy. That's why it's always a good idea to cut the fat when you can.

Frying, sautéing, and basting with butter add unnecessary fat and calories to your dishes. If you're used to adding butter and oil, try cutting back to half the amount the recipe calls for, increasing only as you need to—like adding a little oil so the onions don't burn.

On the other hand, baking, steaming, and boiling use far fewer calories than anything involving oil. Grilling and roasting impart a lot of flavor but not necessarily calories.

Beware of creams and cheeses. Jeanette is the author of three books on cheese, and she adores all things dairy, but she knows to use them sparingly (unless she's making something like macaroni and cheese). Cheese is one of the most calorie-dense and sodium-laden foods on the planet. If you can reduce the amount in a recipe, you reduce the calories immensely, too. Using high-quality, artisan cheeses means you can use just a little bit for a whole lot of flavor.

✪ Mexican Corn on the Cob

This flavorful corn on the cob is sweet yet spicy.

Yield:	Prep time:	Cook time:	Serving size:
6 corn cobs	5 minutes	5 minutes	1 corn cob

Each serving has:				
278 calories	24g fat	13g saturated fat	57mg cholesterol	671mg sodium
2.9g sugar	17g carbohydrates	2.2g fiber	2.4g protein	

6 ears fresh corn, husk and silk removed

3 TB. unsalted butter

3 TB. mayonnaise

12 TB. cream cheese with red peppers

3 tsp. smoked Spanish paprika

$1^1/_2$ tsp. cumin

Sea salt

Fresh ground black pepper

1. Bring a large pot of water to boil over medium high heat. Add corn ears, and boil for 5 minutes or until tender. Remove ears from water, and drain.

2. Onto each ear, spread $1^1/_2$ teaspoons butter, followed by $1^1/_2$ teaspoons mayonnaise, followed by 2 tablespoons cheese.

3. Sprinkle each with $^1/_2$ teaspoon smoked Spanish paprika and $^1/_4$ teaspoon cumin.

4. Season with sea salt and black pepper, and serve.

 FOOD FOR THOUGHT

Traditionally, this recipe is made with Oaxacan cheese or queso blanco and then sprinkled with chili powder, but it's faster to use a cream cheese that's already flavored with hot chiles. Boursin Red Chili Pepper Gornay Cheese or a pimento cheese with jalapeños works well.

⊕ ✿ Stuffed Bell Peppers

Even though these stuffed bell peppers are vegan, they're quite savory and hearty with just a touch of cranberry sweetness.

Yield:	Prep time:	Cook time:	Serving size:
6 stuffed peppers	15 minutes	1 hour, 30 minutes	1 stuffed pepper

Each serving has:				
401 calories	3g fat	0.5g saturated fat	0mg cholesterol	11mg sodium
7g sugar	74g carbohydrates	24g fiber	20g protein	

1 TB. extra-virgin olive oil	1 (14.5-oz.) can diced tomatoes, with juice
¹/₂ large yellow onion, diced (about 1 cup)	¹/₂ cup cooked jasmine rice
2 cloves garlic, minced	Sea salt
¹/₂ cup red lentils	Freshly ground black pepper
2 cups water	6 medium green or red bell peppers, tops cut off and ribs and seeds removed
2 bay leaves	
¹/₂ cup dried cranberries	

1. In a medium saucepan over high heat, heat extra-virgin olive oil for 1 minute. Reduce heat to medium-high, add yellow onion and garlic, and sauté for 5 minutes.

2. Add red lentils, water, and bay leaves. Bring to a boil, reduce heat to medium-low, partially cover, and simmer for 10 minutes or until almost all water has been absorbed.

3. Add cranberries and diced tomatoes with juice, and cook for about 10 to 15 more minutes or until water from tomatoes is reduced. Remove bay leaves, and turn off stove.

4. Preheat the oven to 350°F.

5. Stir cooked rice into cooked lentils. Season with sea salt and black pepper. Evenly divide rice-lentil mixture among bell peppers, and top with pepper tops. Place peppers in a 9×13-inch baking dish, and bake for 30 minutes.

Variation: For extra crunch, add 1 or 2 tablespoons toasted almonds to the rice and lentils mixture. Or add 1 or 2 tablespoons chopped kalamata olives for extra flavor. You also can top with grated cheese if you like. Parmesan and chèvre both work well.

☻ Roasted Tomato BLTs

BLTs are delicious, but when you roast the tomatoes, this classic sandwich is taken to a place that's both sweet and salty.

Yield:	Prep time:	Cook time:	Serving size:
2 sandwiches	10 minutes	15 minutes	1 sandwich

Each serving has:				
416 calories	23g fat	5g saturated fat	35mg cholesterol	773mg sodium
6g sugar	37g carbohydrates	5.4g fiber	12.4g protein	

3 slices bacon

4 slices gluten-free bread

2 TB. Basic Mayonnaise (recipe in Chapter 15)

4 large leaves red or green leaf lettuce, cut in $^1/_2$

6 roasted roma tomato halves, sliced

1. In a large, nonstick or cast-iron pan, place bacon slices. Set over high heat, and as soon as bacon begins to sizzle, reduce heat to medium and cook, turning bacon with tongs to cook both sides, for 5 or 6 minutes or bacon until is crispy. Cut each slice in half.

2. Meanwhile, toast bread.

3. Evenly spread Basic Mayonnaise over bread.

4. To assemble, place red lettuce leaves on 2 slices of bread, layer with roma tomatoes, add 3 bacon slice halves to each, and top with remaining slice of bread. Cut sandwiches in half, and serve.

Variation: For an herbal mayonnaise, mix in 1 teaspoon minced parsley, 1 teaspoon minced chives, and 1 clove minced garlic before spreading on the bread.

FOOD FOR THOUGHT

Roasted tomatoes are easy to make, and the resulting flavor is so worth it. Preheat the oven to 350ºF. For 5 pounds fresh roma tomatoes, you'll get 1 quart roasted tomatoes. Core each tomato, slice in half, and squeeze the seeds out of each half. Place tomatoes skin side down in large roasting pan. Drizzle with about $1^1/_2$ teaspoon extra-virgin olive oil, season with about $^1/_2$ teaspoon sea salt and $^1/_2$ teaspoon fresh ground black pepper, and roast for 1 hour or until tomatoes slightly char.

☻ Gluten-Free Meatloaf

This moist and hearty meatloaf has just a touch of garlic. In addition, it packs a protein punch thanks to a secret ingredient—quinoa flakes.

Yield:	Prep time:	Cook time:	Serving size:	
1 (10×5-in.) loaf	10 minutes	60 minutes	1 slice	
Each serving has:				
270 calories	11g fat	4g saturated fat	100mg cholesterol	92mg sodium
1.5g sugar	10g carbohydrates	1.4g fiber	31g protein	

2 lb. ground chuck, veal, and pork mixture

1 medium zucchini, shredded

1 cup quinoa flakes

2 large eggs, lightly beaten

$^1/_2$ medium yellow or white onion, finely diced

2 cloves garlic, minced

1 TB. dried parsley flakes

$1^1/_2$ tsp. cinnamon

Sea salt

Freshly ground black pepper

$1^1/_2$ cups gluten-free ketchup

1. Preheat the oven to 350°F.

2. In a large bowl, combine ground chuck mixture, zucchini, quinoa flakes, eggs, yellow onion, garlic, parsley, cinnamon, sea salt, and black pepper.

3. Using your hands, form mixture into a loaf, and place in a 10×5-inch bread pan. Top with ketchup.

4. Bake for 1 hour. Slice, and serve.

Variation: Meatloaves are great ways to sneak in vegetables. Add $^1/_2$ cup chopped carrots or $^1/_2$ cup chopped spinach or kale. Substitute the new veggies for the zucchini, reduce the meat by $^1/_4$ pound to make exactly same size loaf, or just add extra veggies in for a larger loaf. You can also substitute with ground chicken or turkey to lower the calories. Instead of ketchup, you could use $1^1/_2$ cups spaghetti sauce or barbecue sauce.

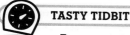 **TASTY TIDBIT**

For an easy tomato sauce, whisk together 1 (6-ounce) can tomato paste, 1 cup water, 1 tablespoon sugar, 1 tablespoon dried parsley flakes, $^1/_2$ teaspoon onion powder, $^1/_2$ teaspoon garlic powder, and sea salt and freshly ground black pepper to taste. Pour over meatloaf in place of the ketchup.

☻ Braised Short Ribs

This hearty meal is a perfect dinner for a slow cooker, and it smells so good while it's cooking, you will not want to wait to eat it!

Yield:	Prep time:	Cook time:	Serving size:
4 or 5 pounds short ribs	15 minutes	8 1/2 hours	about 1 cup or 1/2 pound short ribs

Each serving has:				
594 calories	24.3g fat	8.8g saturated fat	232mg cholesterol	411mg sodium
4.2g sugar	10g carbohydrates	2.8g fiber	77g protein	

3 slices bacon	1 cup red wine
4 or 5 lb. beef short ribs	2 cup beef broth or stock, reduced or no sodium
2 medium yellow onions, diced (about 2 cups)	1 tsp. cinnamon
2 large carrots, peeled and diced (about 1 cup)	1 TB. fresh savory
2 stalks celery, diced (about 1/2 cup)	2 tsp. fresh rosemary
8 oz. white mushrooms, sliced	2 bay leaves
8 oz. baby bella mushrooms, sliced	1/2 tsp. sea salt
4 TB. tomato paste	Freshly ground black pepper

1. Preheat a slow cooker to low.

2. In a large skillet over medium heat, fry bacon. Remove bacon from the skillet, and reserve for another use.

3. Set skillet over high heat, add short ribs, and cook for about 10 minutes or until brown on all sides. Place short ribs in the slow cooker.

4. Add yellow onions to the skillet, and sauté for 2 minutes. Add carrots and celery, and sauté for 2 more minutes. Using a slotted spoon, remove vegetables from the skillet and add to the slow cooker.

5. Add white mushrooms and baby bella mushrooms to the skillet, and sauté for 5 to 8 mintues or until browned. You might need to add a little grapeseed or vegetable oil if bacon grease is all used up by this point. Using a slotted spoon, remove mushrooms from the skillet and add to the slow cooker.

6. Add tomato paste, red wine, beef broth, cinnamon, savory, rosemary, bay leaves, sea salt, and black pepper to the slow cooker. Cover and cook for 8 hours.

7. Using a slotted spoon, remove beef and mushrooms from the slow cooker, and place in large bowl.

8. Remove the bay leaves, place remaining ingredients in a blender or a food processor fitted with a standard S-blade, and pulse until smooth. Pour over beef and mushrooms, and serve.

FOOD FOR THOUGHT

This dish is traditionally served with potatoes, but it also tastes great when served over rice.

☸ Crab Cakes

The best crab cakes taste like crab, not glutenous crumbs or fillers. These crab cakes taste of pure crab and not much else. They're so delicious you'll probably want to double or triple the recipe.

Yield:		Prep time:	Cook time:	Serving size:
4 (4-inch) crab cakes		10 minutes	5 minutes	1 crab cake
Each serving has:				
68 calories	1g fat	0g saturated fat	49mg cholesterol	410mg sodium
3g sugar	9g carbohydrates	0.2g fiber	5g protein	

1 (6-oz.) can lump crabmeat, drained

1/4 cup rice crumbs or gluten-free breadcrumbs

2 TB. yellow onion, minced

1 TB. green bell pepper, minced

1 TB. fresh dill, minced

1 large egg, lightly beaten

2 tsp. Dijon mustard

1 tsp. gluten-free seafood seasoning

1 tsp. fresh lemon juice

Sea salt

2 tsp. corn or canola oil

1. In a large bowl, combine crabmeat, rice crumbs, yellow onion, green bell pepper, dill, egg, Dijon mustard, seafood seasoning, lemon juice, and sea salt. (Mixture will be quite wet but shouldn't fall apart as you work with it. If mixture is too wet, add more rice crumbs 1 teaspoon at at time.) Using your hands, form 4 (4-inch) crab cakes.

2. Heat a large, nonstick or iron skillet over high heat for 1 minute. Wipe or spray with cooking oil, and return to heat for 1 more minute.

3. Place crab cakes into the hot pan, and cook for 2 minutes per side or until brown. Serve immediately.

TASTY TIDBIT

These crab cakes taste great plain, but serving them with a spicy mayo sauce or remoulade sauce takes them up a notch. For 1/3 cup spicy mayo sauce, combine 4 tablespoons mayonnaise, 1 tablespoon diced onion, 1 tablespoon diced green bell pepper, 2 teaspoons Dijon mustard, 1 teaspoon tomato paste, and 1/2 teaspoon smoked paprika.

✪ ◑ *Salmon en Papillote*

Sweet and herbal, this steamed salmon and vegetable dish not only is healthy, its individual packages make for a beautiful presentation.

Yield:	Prep time:	Cook time:	Serving size:	
4 salmon package	15 minutes	15 minutes	1 salmon packages	
Each serving has:				
272 calories	7.6g fat	1.4g saturated fat	0mg cholesterol	28mg sodium
12g sugar	17g carbohydrates	2.4g fiber	41g protein	

1 medium zucchini, thinly sliced

1 medium yellow squash, thinly sliced

1 large carrot, peeled and thinly sliced

1 medium yellow onion, thinly sliced

$^2/_3$ cup lemon juice or juice from $1^1/_2$ lemons

2 TB. fresh parsley, minced

2 TB. fresh thyme, pulled from stalks

3 cloves garlic, minced

2 TB. extra-virgin olive oil

2 TB. honey

Sea salt

Freshly ground black pepper

4 ($^1/_3$-lb.) fresh, boneless salmon fillets

1. Preheat the oven to 425°F. Cut 4 pieces of parchment paper, about 14 to 16 inches in length. Set aside.

2. In a large bowl, combine zucchini, yellow squash, carrot, and yellow onion.

3. In a small bowl, whisk together lemon juice, parsley, thyme, garlic, extra-virgin olive oil, and honey. Season with sea salt and black pepper, and set aside.

4. Lay 1 piece of parchment paper down on your counter or workspace. Place about 1 cup vegetable mixture in the middle, and place 1 salmon fillet on top. Season with sea salt and black pepper, and drizzle 2 tablespoons lemon juice mixture on top. Fold parchment paper so the top and bottom halves meet and then fold over twice to seal. Fold the side edges inward and under so the paper won't unwrap. Repeat with each remaining ingredient and pieces of parchment paper. (You'll have a bit of lemon juice mixture left over. Store in the refrigerator to use for something else.) Place packages on a baking sheet.

5. Bake for 15 minutes. Place packages on individual plates, and serve.

Variation: Feel free to use your favorite vegetables in this recipe. Use fresh asparagus, broccoli, and spinach instead of the zucchini, squash, and carrots, for example. You also can replace the herbs with fresh tarragon, sage, basil, or cilantro—use whatever's in season or in your garden.

❽ Salmon Corn Chowder

The sweetness of fresh corn combines with the delicious meatiness of salmon to create a creamy, tasty soup with just a touch of dill. It's perfect alongside cornbread.

Yield:	Prep time:	Cook time:	Serving size:
12 cups	30 minutes	30 minutes	$1^1/_2$ cups

Each serving has:				
210 calories	4.5g fat	0g saturated fat	0mg cholesterol	270mg sodium
3g sugar	25g carbohydrates	3g fiber	16g protein	

2 medium russet or Idaho potatoes, peeled

2 medium carrots, peeled

1 medium stalk celery, diced

1 medium yellow onion, diced

1 tsp. extra-virgin olive oil

2 TB. cornstarch dissolved in 2 TB. water

1 cup skim milk

1 (32-oz.) pkg. low-sodium chicken or fish stock

2 (6-oz.) cans salmon packed in water, without bones or skin

2 cups corn, freshly shucked or frozen

2 tsp. Old Bay seasoning

Sea salt

Fresh ground black pepper

1 TB. dill, finely minced

1. Place russet potatoes and carrots in a large pot, cover with water, bring to a boil over medium-high heat, and boil for 8 to 10 minutes. Drain potatoes and carrots in a colander, pour cold water over top, and let cool for 5 minutes. Remove potatoes and carrots, and dice.

2. Meanwhile, preheat a large stockpot over medium-high heat for 2 minutes. Lightly coat with olive oil cooking spray, and let heat for 30 more seconds. Add celery and yellow onion, and sauté for 2 or 3 minutes or until onions are translucent.

3. Add extra-virgin olive oil and cornstarch mixture, and whisk for 1 or 2 minutes to create a roux.

4. Add skim milk, whisking it in $^1/_4$ cup at a time.

5. Pour in chicken broth, and add salmon, potatoes, carrots, corn, and Old Bay seasoning. Cook for 5 or 6 minutes. If chowder seems too thin, add more cornstarch, $^1/_2$ teaspoon at a time dissolved in $^1/_2$ teaspoon water. When it thickens to your liking, reduce heat to medium-low, and simmer for at least 10 more minutes. Season with sea salt and black pepper.

6. Add dill 1 minute before serving, stir, and serve.

Variation: This chowder tastes richer if you use cream or crème fraîche instead of skim milk. If you use cream or crème fraîche, reduce the cornstarch to 1 tablespoon mixed with 1 tablespoon water. This recipe also tastes great if you use fresh salmon. Broil a 12-ounce fillet for 5 minutes, remove the bones and skin, and add to chowder.

 TASTY TIDBIT

If you use crème fraîche and you really like the taste of dill, add 1 extra tablespoon minced dill, and mix the dill into the crème fraîche first. Let it marinate for 1 hour to infuse the dill flavor into the crème fraîche.

❽ Broiled Tilapia with Cranberry Honey Mustard

This delicate white fish has a kick of lemon and spice. The accompanying cranberry honey mustard adds an extra layer or two of fresh flavor.

Yield:	Prep time:	Cook time:	Serving size:
6 fillets plus 1¹/₂ cups sauce	15 minutes	30 minutes	1 fillet plus 2 tablespoons sauce

Each serving has:				
210 calories	2.5g fat	1g saturated fat	75mg cholesterol	240mg sodium
10g sugar	15g carbohydrates	2g fiber	31g protein	

1 cup frozen or fresh cranberries	1 tsp. Cajun seasoning
1 cup orange juice	Sea salt
Zest of 1 orange	Fresh ground black pepper
1 tsp. vanilla extract	1 medium lemon, sliced thin
6 (¹/₃-lb.) tilapia fillets (about 2 lb.)	3 TB. honey
2 tsp. fresh dill, minced	3 TB. Dijon mustard
2 tsp. fresh parsley, minced	2 tsp. fresh squeezed lemon juice
1 tsp. Old Bay seasoning	

1. In a medium saucepan over medium-high heat, combine cranberries, orange juice, orange zest, and vanilla extract. Cook for 5 to 10 minutes or until sauce starts to boil and cranberries start to pop.

2. Reduce heat to medium-low, and cook, stirring occasionally, for about 15 to 20 minutes or until thickened and slightly reduced.

3. Meanwhile, preheat the broiler to high.

4. Place tilapia in a shallow baking dish, and sprinkle with dill, parsley, Old Bay seasoning, Cajun seasoning, sea salt, and black pepper. Lay a few lemon slices in the middle of each fillet.

5. Broil fillets for 8 to 10 minutes or until cooked through but still moist.

6. Remove sauce from heat, and whisk in honey and Dijon mustard.

7. Drizzle tilapia with lemon juice, top with cranberry honey mustard, and serve.

> **FOOD FOR THOUGHT**
>
> Tilapia is raised in many American fish farms, and according to the Monterrey Bay Aquarium Seafood Watch, the fish is a "best choice," meaning it is one of the most sustainable seafood choices you can make.

⊗ *Arroz con Pollo*

This Puerto Rican chicken and rice dish is like a less soupy version of chicken and rice soup, but with a kick of spice and a dollop of umami thanks to the olives.

Yield:	Prep time:	Cook time:	Serving size:
8 cups	60 minutes	1 hour, 30 minutes	2 cups

Each serving has:			
528 calories	15.7g fat	3.4g saturated fat	101mg cholesterol 1074mg sodium
9.8g sugar	55g carbohydrates	5.2g fiber	40.4g protein

1 cup brown basmati rice

$1^1/_2$ cups chicken stock

3 tsp. extra-virgin olive oil

1 medium onion, roughly chopped

1 green bell pepper, ribs and seeds removed, and roughly chopped

2 medium plum tomatoes, roughly chopped

4 cloves garlic

5 TB. fresh cilantro, minced

1 tsp. cumin

2 large boneless chicken breasts (about $1^1/_4$ lb.), diced

Sea salt

Freshly ground black pepper

1 large tomato, chopped

1 cup frozen or fresh peas

1 cup kalamata, green pimento, or your choice olives, pitted and chopped

2 cups chicken stock

$^1/_2$ tsp. turmeric

$^1/_2$ tsp. sweet Spanish paprika

2 tsp. honey

1 tsp. balsamic vinegar

1. In a medium saucepan over medium heat, cook brown basmati rice in chicken stock according to the package directions.

2. Meanwhile, heat a large saucepan over high heat for 2 minutes. Add 2 teaspoons extra-virgin olive oil, reduce heat to medium-high, and heat for 30 seconds.

3. Add onion, and sauté for 5 minutes. Reduce heat to low, and cook, stirring occasionally, for about 20 to 30 minutes.

4. When onion has caramelized, increase heat to medium-high, and add green bell pepper, plum tomatoes, garlic, 4 tablespoons cilantro, and cumin. Sauté for about 5 to 8 minutes or until all vegetables are cooked.

5. In a food processor fitted with a standard blade, purée onion mixture for about 1 minute. (Makes 2 cups sofrito, but you only need 1 cup for this dish, so freeze 1 cup for up to 3 months or use to season tacos or other dishes.)

6. Heat a large pot over medium-high heat for 2 minutes. Add remaining 1 teaspoon extra-virgin olive oil, and heat for 1 minute.

7. Season chicken with sea salt and black pepper, add to the pot, and sauté for about 5 minutes or until no longer pink.

8. Add tomato, peas, and olives, and sauté for about 3 minutes or until cooked.

9. Add remaining chicken stock, cooked rice, 1 cup sofrito, turmeric, and sweet Spanish paprika. Reduce heat to medium, and cook, stirring frequently, for 5 minutes.

10. Season with sea salt, and taste.

11. Add honey, balsamic vinegar, and remaining 1 tablespoon cilantro. Cook for 1 more minute, and serve.

 FOOD FOR THOUGHT

Traditional arroz con pollo uses green olives stuffed with pimentos, but use whatever olives you like best. (Jeanette likes a mixture of green and kalamata olives.) The dish also often calls for pigeon peas, which you can find in the frozen section of Latin markets. Or use regular peas or even edamame. One very important nutritional point: if you use homemade stock, you can reduce the amount of sodium dramatically.

✪ Chicken Almondine with Lemon Green Beans

Almonds give these chicken breasts a bit of crunch and flavor, and when served alongside these tangy green beans, you've got a fantastic meal.

Yield:	Prep time:	Cook time:	Serving size:
4 chicken breasts and 3 cups green beans	20 minutes	30 minutes	1 chicken breast with $^3/_4$ cup green beans

Each serving has:				
220 calories	6g fat	.75g saturated fat	66mg cholesterol	111mg sodium
2g sugar	12g carbohydrates	5g fiber	30g protein	

$^1/_4$ cup toasted, slivered, unsalted almonds

1 TB. All-Purpose Gluten-Free Flour Blend (recipe in Chapter 18)

$^1/_2$ tsp. sea salt

$^1/_2$ tsp. fresh ground black pepper

$^1/_2$ tsp. Cajun seasoning

4 ($^1/_4$-lb.) boneless, skinless chicken breasts, pounded to $^1/_2$-in. thickness

1 lb. fresh green beans, ends removed

Zest of 1 large lemon (about 2 or 3 tsp.)

Juice of $^1/_2$ large lemon (about 1 TB.)

Sea salt

1. In a food processor fitted with a standard S-blade, grind $^1/_8$ cup almonds for 1 or 2 minutes until a fine powder.

2. In a medium bowl, combine ground almonds, All-Purpose Gluten-Free Flour Blend, sea salt, black pepper, and Cajun seasoning.

3. Dredge chicken breasts in almond mixture, and set aside.

4. Heat a large, nonstick or cast-iron skillet over high heat for 2 minutes. Lightly coat with olive oil cooking spray, and heat for 30 more seconds. Reduce heat to medium-high, add chicken breasts, and sauté for 3 minutes per side or until golden brown and no pink remains. Remove from heat.

5. Bring a large pot of water to a boil over medium-high heat. Add green beans, and blanch for 1 minute. Remove beans from water, add to a large bowl, and toss with lemon zest, lemon juice, sea salt, and more black pepper.

6. Sprinkle remaining $1/8$ cup almonds over chicken, dividing evenly among breasts, and serve alongside green beans.

 FOOD FOR THOUGHT

Not every meal has to have a protein, a veggie, and a starch, but if you like to have a starch with your dinner, these chicken breasts and green beans go quite well with our Rice Pilaf (recipe in Chapter 16).

Chicken, Cauliflower, and Potato Curry

Creamy and coconutty, this savory, Thai-style curry has just a touch of heat.

Yield:	Prep time:	Cook time:	Serving size:
6½ to 7 cups	15 minutes	45 minutes	1 cup

Each serving has:				
215 calories	8.7g fat	6.2g saturated fat	32mg cholesterol	580mg sodium
5g sugar	20g carbohydrates	2g fiber	16g protein	

3 medium Yukon gold potatoes (about 1 lb.)

2 tsp. coconut oil

1 medium yellow onion, diced (about 1 cup)

2 boneless, skinless chicken breasts, extra fat removed and cubed (about 1 lb.)

1 medium head cauliflower, cut into florets (about 1½ lb.)

2 (13.5-oz.) cans reduced-fat coconut milk

1 TB. gluten-free Thai red curry paste

1 TB. gluten-free Thai fish sauce

1 TB. tamari

1 TB. sugar

1 TB. cornstarch

2 TB. water

1. Using a fork, poke holes in Yukon gold potatoes, and place in a microwave-safe dish. Cook on high for 2 minutes. Peel and dice.

2. Heat a large pot over high heat for 2 minutes. Add coconut oil, and heat for 2 more minutes.

3. Add yellow onion, reduce heat to medium-high, and sauté for 1 minute.

4. Add chicken breasts, and sauté for 5 minutes or until almost completely cooked.

5. Add potatoes and cauliflower, and sauté for 2 minutes.

6. Add coconut milk, Thai red curry paste, Thai fish sauce, tamari, and sugar. Reduce heat to medium, and cook for about 20 to 25 minutes or until cauliflower is tender and flavors have melded.

7. In a small bowl, whisk cornstarch into water to dissolve. Add to curry, and cook for 5 minutes or until coconut sauce has thickened enough to coat the back of a spoon.

8. Serve over rice, garnish with chopped cilantro leaves if desired.

 GLUTEN GAFFE

There's a big difference between reduced-fat and regular coconut cream. The taste is similar, but the calories and fat are higher in the regular version.

ⓥ Curried Sweet Potato Soup

Sweet and creamy, this lentil and sweet potato soup stars garlic and ginger with just a touch of heat.

Yield:	Prep time:	Cook time:	Serving size:
6 cups	20 minutes	40 minutes	1¹/₂ cups

Each serving has:				
245 calories	6g fat	3.8g saturated fat	0mg cholesterol	792mg sodium
7g sugar	34g carbohydrates	11.5g fiber	13g protein	

2 tsp. coconut oil

1 large yellow onion, diced

6 cloves garlic, minced

1 (1-in.) piece fresh ginger, peeled and minced

1 cup red lentils, well rinsed

4 cups vegetable stock

1 large sweet potato (at least 1 lb.), peeled and diced

2 cups coconut milk

2 TB. red curry paste

Sea salt

Freshly ground white pepper

3 TB. fresh cilantro, minced

1. In a large pot over medium-high heat, heat coconut oil. Add yellow onion, and sauté for about 5 minutes or until onion turns translucent.

2. Add garlic and ginger, and sauté for 1 minute. Add red lentils, and sauté for 1 minute.

3. Add 2 cups vegetable stock, reduce heat to medium, cover, and cook, stirring occasionally, for 15 minutes or until lentils are almost done.

4. Add sweet potato, remaining 2 cups vegetable stock, and coconut milk. Cook, stirring frequently, for 10 to 15 more minutes or until sweet potatoes are soft. Stir in red curry paste, season with sea salt and pepper, and add cilantro.

5. In a blender or a food processor fitted with a standard S-blade, purée soup until smooth. Serve, garnished with extra cilantro.

Variation: Add extra curry paste if you like it hotter.

 FOOD FOR THOUGHT

It's easier to purée the soup if you have an immersion blender, which enables you to purée the soup right in the pot.

Cornbread and Sausage Stuffing

This savory and herby stuffing tastes a little bit like a sausage and corn biscuit sandwich.

Yield:	Prep time:	Cook time:	Serving size:
10 cups	15 minutes	1 hour, 30 minutes	$^1/_2$ cup

Each serving has:				
239 calories	17.4g fat	9g saturated fat	106mg cholesterol	300mg sodium
2g sugar	15.6g carbohydrates	1.5g fiber	6.6g protein	

1 tsp. canola oil

$^1/_4$ lb. bulk breakfast sausage

1 medium yellow onion, diced

1 stalk celery, diced

$^1/_2$ batch Cornbread (recipe in Chapter 18), left out to dry overnight

$^1/_3$ cup fresh parsley, minced

1 TB. fresh sage, minced

1 TB. fresh thyme, minced

$^1/_2$ tsp. sea salt

$^1/_2$ tsp. nutmeg

$^1/_2$ tsp. freshly ground black pepper

2 cups no-salt-added chicken broth or stock

2 large eggs, lightly beaten

2 TB. unsalted butter

1. Preheat the oven to 350°F.

2. Heat a medium saucepan over medium-high heat for 1 minute. Add canola oil, and heat for 1 minute.

3. Add breakfast sausage, cook for about 5 to 8 minutes or until no longer pink.

4. Add yellow onion, and sauté for 2 more minutes.

5. Add celery, and cook for 1 or 2 minutes.

6. In a large bowl, crumble Cornbread. Add parsley, sage, thyme, sea salt, nutmeg, and black pepper. Add cooked sausage, onions, and celery, and stir in chicken broth and eggs. Pour stuffing into 10-cup casserole dish, and dot with 2 tablespoons unsalted butter.

7. Bake for 60 minutes or until slightly browned on top and puffed up like a soufflé. Serve immediately.

Variation: You can replace the pork breakfast sausage with chicken or turkey sausage. Or you can eliminate the sausage all together if you want.

☻ Apple and Raisin Stuffing

Sweet with apples and raisins, this savory, herbal stuffing is perfect for Thanksgiving.

Yield:	Prep time:	Cook time:	Serving size:
10 cups	2 minutes	30 minutes	1 cup

Each serving has:				
133 calories	6.2g fat	1.8g saturated fat	6mg cholesterol	266mg sodium
6.9g sugar	17.8g carbohydrates	2.1g fiber	1.4g protein	

$1^1/_2$ tsp. plus 1 TB. canola oil	$^1/_3$ cup fresh parsley, minced
1 medium yellow onion, diced	1 TB. fresh sage, minced
1 stalk celery, diced	1 TB. fresh thyme, minced
1 medium Gala apple, peeled, cored, and diced	$^1/_2$ tsp. sea salt
$^1/_2$ cup raisins	$^1/_2$ tsp. freshly ground black pepper
5 cups cubed, gluten-free bread, dried overnight	2 cups no-salt-added vegetable or chicken broth
	2 TB. unsalted butter

1. Preheat the oven to 350°F.

2. Heat a medium saucepan over medium-high heat for 1 minute. Add $1^1/_2$ teaspoons canola oil, and heat for 1 minute.

3. Add yellow onion, and sauté for 2 minutes.

4. Add celery, and cook for 1 or 2 minutes.

5. Add Gala apple and raisins, and sauté for 1 more minute.

6. In a large bowl, toss bread cubes, parsley, sage, thyme, sea salt, and black pepper. Toss with cooked vegetables and fruits, and stir in vegetable broth and remaining 1 tablespoon canola oil. Pour into 10-cup casserole dish, and dot with 2 tablespoons unsalted butter.

7. Bake for 60 minutes or until slightly browned on top.

Variation: This stuffing tastes even better when you add 2 eggs. Add them when you add the broth.

🌱 ☣ **Rice Pilaf**

This easy rice pilaf is very fragrant with just a touch of sweetness.

Yield:	Prep time:	Cook time:	Serving size:
4 cups	2 minutes	45 minutes	$^1/_2$ cup

Each serving has:				
126 calories	2.6g fat	0g saturated fat	0mg cholesterol	7mg sodium
3.6g sugar	24g carbohydrates	1.7g fiber	2.2g protein	

1 tsp. cinnamon	2 cups no-salt-added vegetable stock
$^1/_2$ tsp. celery seeds	$^1/_4$ cup slivered, toasted almonds
1 TB. canola oil	$^1/_4$ cup golden raisins or dried cranberries
1 medium yellow onion, diced (about 1 cup)	1 tsp. agave syrup or honey
1 medium carrot, peeled and diced (about $^1/_3$ cup)	$^1/_2$ tsp. apple cider vinegar
2 cloves garlic, minced	Sea salt
1 cup brown rice	Freshly ground black pepper

1. Heat a medium saucepan over high heat. Add cinnamon and celery seeds, and toast for about 1 minute.

2. Add canola oil, and heat for 1 minute. Reduce heat to medium.

3. Add yellow onion, carrot, and garlic, and sauté for about 5 minutes or until softened.

4. Increase heat to high, and add brown rice, vegetable stock, almonds, raisins, agave syrup, and apple cider vinegar. Bring to a boil, reduce heat to medium-low, cover, and simmer, stirring frequently, for about 30 minutes or until all liquid has been absorbed.

5. Season with salt and pepper, and serve.

Variation: To give this dish a more vibrant, yellow color, add $^1/_2$ teaspoon turmeric.

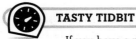 **TASTY TIDBIT**

If you have a rice cooker, you can steam the vegetables, rice, stock, almonds, raisins, agave, and apple cider vinegar in it for 35 minutes.

✪ Basic Risotto

A touch of garlic and a little white wine elevate this creamy and cheesy risotto dish to new levels of deliciousness.

Yield:	Prep time:	Cook time:	Serving size:
4 cups	2 minutes	30 minutes	1/2 cup

Each serving has:				
269 calories	7.7g fat	3g saturated fat	15mg cholesterol	108mg sodium
0g sugar	40g carbohydrates	1.4g fiber	9g protein	

2 TB. extra-virgin olive oil

1/4 medium yellow onion, diced (1/4 cup)

2 cloves garlic, minced

2 cups arborio rice

1/2 cup Pinot Grigio or your favorite white wine

3 cups no-salt-added chicken stock

1 cup low-fat ricotta cheese

1/4 cup grated Parmigiano-Reggiano cheese

Sea salt

Freshly ground white pepper

1. Heat a large pot over high heat for 1 minute. Add extra-virgin olive oil, and heat for 2 minutes.

2. Add yellow onion and garlic, reduce heat to medium-high, and sauté for 5 minutes.

3. Add arborio rice, and cook, stirring constantly, for 2 minutes or until rice is shiny. (This hardens the outer starch.)

4. Pour in wine, and bring to a simmer.

5. Add chicken stock, about 1/2 cup at a time, and cook, stirring constantly, for about 30 minutes or until rice is cooked and creamy. Rice will be tender but not mushy.

6. Stir in ricotta cheese and Parmigiano-Reggiano cheese, season with sea salt and white pepper, and serve.

 TASTY TIDBIT

To make this a traditional risotto Milanese, add a pinch of saffron threads. To do this, bring the stock to a boil, and add the saffron a thread at a time until it becomes nicely yellow and fragrant. Only add the saffron a thread at a time; otherwise, it can be overpowering and you'll use too much.

CHAPTER 17

Perfect Pastas

At one time, the thought of never eating pasta again probably left you feeling discouraged. Rest assured, you can still eat pasta. And your choices are increasing, as more manufacturers are creating gluten-free pastas. Even if you can't find the right premade pasta for your dish, you can easily make your own from scratch.

In this chapter, we show you how to do it by covering the equipment you'll need, sharing some pasta-making tips, and providing great recipes including ravioli, gnocchi, and pierogi. You'll be making from-scratch pastas in no time!

In This Chapter

- Making your own pasta
- Tips for getting pasta just right
- Fun and flavorful pasta recipes

Essential Equipment

With a food processor or a stand-alone mixer, you can whip up pasta dough in minutes. If you don't have either one of these, mixing it by hand works, too. We have found that a pasta maker—either a stand-alone, hand-crank model or a pasta-making attachment for your standing mixer—really makes the job easier. Jeanette's Atlas hand-crank pasta-maker, which she found at an Italian grocery store, is one of her favorite kitchen accoutrements.

If you love pasta and miss not having great ravioli and fresh pasta, consider investing in a pasta maker. We both love the hand-crank kind and have heard automatic pasta makers do not handle gluten-free dough as well as the hand-crank versions.

If you don't have a pasta maker, you can use a rolling pin, which takes some strength and patience, but still delivers delicious results.

 TASTY TIDBIT

Thomas Jefferson brought the first pasta machine to the United States in 1789. He didn't call pasta "pasta" but "macaroni."

Pasta-Making Tips

A pasta maker has settings from 1 to 9, with the lower the number the thicker the pasta, and the higher the number the thinner the pasta. Because gluten-free pasta dough tends to be more delicate than its glutenous cousins, keep your pasta maker set at 5 or below.

Also, because of the dough's delicacy, you might want to have an assistant either feed the dough into the machine or catch it as it comes out, so you can have longer strips. But if you're working alone, use smaller amounts so you can better handle it.

Before making your first batch of dough, you might want to watch some gluten-free pasta-making videos on the internet. Just do a search on Google or YouTube for "making fresh gluten-free pasta." Or you might take a class to see how pasta is made by hand. Some gluten-free pasta classes are available, but even a regular class can help you understand the technique. However, if you do take a glutenous class, do *not* eat the samples.

After you make your fresh pasta, let it dry for at least 2 hours. If you don't plan to cook it immediately after drying, refrigerate or freeze it. You can refrigerate fresh pastas for up to a week or freeze it for up to 3 months. When you dry your pasta, hang it on pasta drying racks, drape long noodles over the edge of very large bowls, or lay them out on cookie sheets. You can also dry fresh pasta in a food dehydrator.

When cooking pasta, whether fresh or store-bought, use a large pot so the pasta has space to spread out so it doesn't stick together and get clumpy. A pot that holds 4 or 5 quarts of water is usually sufficient for one package of pasta, or enough fresh pasta for your family's meal.

It's good to add salt to the pasta cooking water. Salt raises the boiling temperature slightly, which may cook your pasta faster, and it also flavors the pasta noodles a bit. Consider adding 1 or 2 tablespoons salt to 4 or 5 quarts water.

Also, stir the pasta constantly for the first 1 or 2 minutes of boiling so it doesn't stick together. Then, stir occasionally until it's cooked.

For perfect, *al dente* (to the tooth) pasta, use the minimal amount of time recommended on the package or the recipe and then test a piece. If it's softer but still has a little chew to it, it's done. (Of course, if you like your pasta softer, feel free to cook it longer.) Drain but reserve $1/2$ cup water for your sauce. This water will help the sauce better adhere to the noodles, as the starch in the water adds some natural stickiness.

TASTY TIDBIT

Most gluten-free pasta recipes call for eggs. If you don't want to use eggs, flaxseeds are a great substitute, or you can use vegan egg replacers or chia seeds. See Chapter 3 for more on these and other substitutions.

✪ Basic Gluten-Free Pasta Noodles

Use this recipe for spaghetti, fettuccine, lasagna, and even raviolis and stuffed pastas. It's versatile, so it can be a good building block recipe for all your favorite pasta sauces!

Yield:	Prep time:	Dry time:	Serving size:
1 cup pasta	30 minutes	30 to 60 minutes	$1/4$ cup

Each serving has:				
309 calories	1g fat	0g saturated fat	41mg cholesterol	475mg sodium
3g sugar	64g carbohydrates	0g fiber	6.8g protein	

2 cups gluten-free flour	$1/2$ cup water
1 tsp. sea salt	1 large egg
1 tsp. xanthan gum	

1. In a food processor fitted with a standard blade, process gluten-free flour, sea salt, xanthan gum, water, and egg for about 3 minutes or until a smooth dough forms. Scrape dough out of the food processor bowl and turn out onto a clean, lightly floured surface.

2. Knead dough by hand for about 10 minutes or until it's elastic to the touch. You might need to flour your hands as you work the dough.

3. Place kneaded dough in a bowl, cover with a towel or plastic wrap, and let dough rest at room temperature for at least 20 minutes.

4. While dough is resting, clean up flour mess and set up pasta machine. Adjust the machine setting to 1 or the lowest and widest setting.

5. Divide dough into 8 pieces. Flatten 1 piece into about $1/4$ inch thickness, and guide it into the pasta machine, slowly cranking it through. Fold the dough into thirds, and run it through the machine again, still on the first setting, with the folded edges perpendicular to the machine. Then run the pasta through a third time, without folding it.

6. Set the machine to setting 2, and roll pasta through the machine.

7. Set the machine to 3, and roll pasta through the machine again.

8. Set the machine to 4, and roll pasta through the machine once more.

9. Set the machine to 5, and roll pasta through the machine a final time.

10. Place finished pasta on a baking sheet that's been dusted with flour. After all pasta has been rolled into sheets, cut it by hand using a sharp knife or a pizza cutter or gently roll the sheets through the cutting edge of the machine.

11. Let pasta dry on the dusted cookie sheets, hang them on a pasta tree, or lay them over the rims of large bowls for at least 30 to 60 minutes before using. If not using after drying, store in refrigerator in a covered container for up to 1 week.

12. To cook, bring a large pot of salted water to boil, add pasta, and boil until al dente. The wider the pasta, the longer it takes to cook. For narrow spaghetti strands, it takes about 3 minutes. For wider noodles, it can take 4 to 6 minutes.

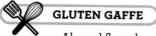

GLUTEN GAFFE

Almond flour does not work well for homemade gluten-free pasta.

☸ Spaghetti with Marinara and Meatballs

This spaghetti dish features tomato sauce with a hint of garlic and lots of sweet basil, and savory meatballs that have just a hint of garlic and onion.

Yield:	Prep time:	Cook time:	Serving size:
8 cups pasta, and 6 cups sauce, 24 meatballs	30 minutes	45 minutes	1 cup pasta, $^1/_2$ cup sauce, and 4 meatballs

Each serving has:				
467 calories	10g fat	2g saturated fat	34mg cholesterol	150mg sodium
11g sugar	69g carbohydrates	4g fiber	18g protein	

1 lb. ground veal, pork, and ground chuck mixture	$^1/_4$ tsp. freshly ground black pepper
$^1/_2$ cup gluten-free panko breadcrumbs	1 (16-oz.) box gluten-free spaghetti
1 large egg, lightly whisked	1 TB. extra-virgin olive oil
1 small yellow onion, finely diced (about $^1/_2$ cup)	1 medium yellow onion, diced
1 clove garlic, finely minced	2 cloves garlic, smashed
2 tsp. gluten-free Italian seasoning blend	1 (28-oz.) can crushed tomatoes
$^1/_2$ tsp. cinnamon	1 (6-oz.) can tomato paste
$^1/_4$ tsp. plus 1 or 2 TB. sea salt	$^3/_4$ cup Sangiovese, Chianti, or other red wine
	1 TB. sugar (optional)
	1 TB. fresh basil, minced

1. Preheat the oven to 350°F.

2. In a large bowl, combine ground veal mixture, panko breadcrumbs, egg, small yellow onion, minced garlic, 1 teaspoon Italian seasoning blend, cinnamon, $^1/_4$ teaspoon sea salt, and $^1/_4$ teaspoon black pepper by hand until well mixed. Wet your hands, and form meat mixture into 24 golf ball–size meatballs.

3. Place meatballs on a nonstick cooking sheet. Bake for 30 minutes or until no longer pink in the center.

4. Meanwhile, in a large pot over high heat, bring 4 or 5 quarts water and remaining 1 or 2 tablespoons sea salt to a rapid boil. Add spaghetti, and cook according to package directions.

5. Heat a medium pot over high heat for 1 minute. Add extra-virgin olive oil, and heat for 30 seconds. Add medium yellow onion and smashed garlic, reduce heat to medium, and cook for 5 minutes or until onion is translucent.

6. Add tomatoes, tomato paste, red wine, sugar (if using), and remaining 1 teaspoon Italian seasoning blend, and season with more sea salt and freshly ground black pepper. Reduce heat to medium, and stir occasionally until sauce comes to a boil. Then reduce heat to low, and continue cooking until your meatballs and pasta are finished.

7. Drain cooked pasta, and remove meatballs from the oven. Remove sauce from heat, stir in fresh basil, and remove garlic.

8. Toss pasta with sauce and meatballs, and serve topped with grated Italian cheese such as Grana Padano.

Variation: If you don't like veal or pork, you can use all ground chuck. Or substitute ground turkey or ground chicken instead. You'll reduce the calories and fat.

 TASTY TIDBIT

To smash the garlic cloves, place them on a cutting board, set the blade of a chef's knife horizontally on top of them, parallel to the cutting board. Press down on the knife blade with your hand, being careful to avoid the sharp edge. Smashing garlic releases its essential oils, and when you sauté and cook smashed garlic in the sauce, it adds a great garlic flavor. By removing it before serving the sauce, you get a sauce with just the right hint of garlic without any actual garlic chunks in the sauce.

✪ Potato Gnocchi

Light and pillowy, these potato gnocchi are divine tossed with a little butter and fresh herbs.

Yield:	Prep time:	Cook time:	Serving size:
about 90 gnocchi	15 minutes	75 minutes	22 gnocchi

Each serving has:				
284 calories	2g fat	1g saturated fat	41mg cholesterol	474mg sodium
2g sugar	60g carbohydrates	8g fiber	6g protein	

5 or 6 medium Yukon gold potatoes (1^1/$_2$ lb.)	1 large egg
1^1/$_2$ cups gluten-free flour	^{1}/$_2$ tsp. xanthan gum
	^{1}/$_2$ tsp. sea salt

1. Preheat the oven to 350°F.

2. Using a fork, poke holes in Yukon gold potatoes. Place on a baking sheet, and bake for 45 minutes.

3. Let potatoes cool for 10 minutes, peel, and roughly chop.

4. Lightly flour the baking sheet. You'll use it again.

5. In a food processor fitted with a standard S blade, purée potatoes. When completely mashed, add flour, egg, xanthan gum, and sea salt. Pulse a few times—for about 30 to 60 seconds—until dough is completely combined.

6. With your hands wet or lightly floured, roll dough into 5 or 6 balls. Roll each ball so it's a 1-inch cylinder, about 10 inches long. Slice cylinder into ^{1}/$_2$-inch pieces, and roll each piece into an oval-shape dumpling about 1 to 1^1/$_2$ inches long. Press the back of a fork around each dumpling to create grooves, and set shaped dumplings on the baking sheet.

7. Bring a large pot of salted water to boil over high heat. Add gnocchi in 2 or 3 batches, and bring water back to a boil. When gnocchi rise to the top of water, remove and place in a colander to drain.

8. Toss with your choice sauce, and serve immediately.

FOOD FOR THOUGHT

The word *gnocchi* is derived from either the Italian word *nocchio*, which means "knot of wood," or *nocca*, which means "knuckle."

⊗ Cheese Ravioli

Creamy and cheesy with just a touch of basil and parsley, these fresh homemade ravioli are delicious.

Yield:	Prep time:	Cook time:	Serving size:
40 raviolis	15 minutes	15 minutes	10 raviolis

Each serving has:				
357 calories	4.2g fat	2.4g saturated fat	51mg cholesterol	842mg sodium
0g sugar	64.8g carbohydrates	0g fiber	11.7g protein	

1 cup low-fat, part-skim ricotta cheese	1 batch Basic Gluten-Free Pasta Noodles (recipe earlier in this chapter), rolled to number 4 or 5 thickness on pasta machine in sheets at least 3 or 4 in. wide
¹/₄ cup grated Parmigiano-Reggiano cheese	
6 fresh basil leaves	
2 TB. fresh parsley, minced	

1. In a food processor fitted with a standard blade, pulse together ricotta cheese, Parmigiano-Reggiano cheese, basil, and parsley for about 2 minutes or until well combined.

2. Cut rough edges from Basic Gluten-Free Pasta Noodles so sheets are even. (Use rough edges for noodles for soup or other use, or discard.) Dust a counter or a cookie sheet with flour, and using a knife, cut sheets into 2×4-inch pieces.

3. Fill a small bowl with water and set near your workspace.

4. To make ravioli, place ¹/₂ teaspoon filling in the middle of the bottom half of 1 piece of pasta dough. Wet your finger in water and run it around edges of pasta piece. Fold pasta in half, using your fingers to press and seal ravioli. Repeat with remaining pasta and filling. When all raviolis are formed, let sit for 30 minutes to rest.

5. Bring large pot of salted water to boil over high heat. Add raviolis, and boil for about 3 to 5 minutes or until al dente. Raviolis are done when they float to the surface.

TASTY TIDBIT

If, as you're filling and sealing the dough, your ravioli isn't as neat or pretty as you want, use a knife to remove any excess dough.

☷ Meat Pierogi

Tender yet slightly chewy, these savory dumplings offer a delicious, meaty flavor.

Yield:	Prep time:	Cook time:	Serving size:
32 pierogi	45 minutes	10 minutes	8 pierogi

Each serving has:				
482 calories	9.3g fat	4.9g saturated fat	75mg cholesterol	163mg sodium
1.7g sugar	82g carbohydrates	0g fiber	12.7g protein	

$^1/_2$ lb. ground sirloin	$2^1/_2$ cups gluten-free flour
Sea salt	2 tsp. xanthan gum
Freshly ground black pepper	$^1/_2$ cup 2 percent milk
Pinch cinnamon	$^1/_2$ cup heavy cream
Pinch nutmeg	1 large egg, lightly beaten
$^1/_2$ cup low- or no-sodium beef broth or stock	1 tsp. apple cider vinegar
1 TB. fresh parsley, minced	

1. Heat a medium saucepan over medium-high heat for 2 minutes. Season ground sirloin with sea salt, black pepper, cinnamon, and nutmeg, and add to the saucepan. Sauté on both sides for about 5 minutes or until no longer red.

2. In a food processor fitted with a standard blade, pulse sirloin, beef broth, and parsley for about 5 minutes or until meat "dough" forms. Remove dough from the food processor, place in a small bowl, cover with plastic wrap, and refrigerate until ready to stuff pierogi.

3. In a large bowl, sift together flour, xanthan gum, and pinch sea salt. Pour in milk, heavy cream, egg, and apple cider vinegar, and stir until combined.

4. Using your hands, gently knead until dough is one smooth, slightly sticky ball.

5. Lightly oil a silicone baking sheet or piece of parchment paper. Place $^1/_4$ of dough in middle, and using a lightly oiled rolling pin, roll dough to $^1/_8$-inch thickness.

6. Use a $3^1/_2$-inch round cookie cutter to slice dough into individual pierogi.

7. Remove filling from the refrigerator, and place 1 rounded teaspoon in center of each dumpling. Fold over dough to create a half-circle, and use your fingers to press and seal pierogi closed.

8. Bring a large pot of salted water to a boil over medium-high heat. Add pierogi, and boil for about 5 minutes or until they float to the surface.

FOOD FOR THOUGHT

Pierogi are filled Polish dumplings. After they're boiled, they're traditionally fried in butter and served with a side of sour cream. You also could fry them in bacon and onions.

CHAPTER 18

Bountiful Breads

Few things smell better than baking bread. And just because you've ditched the wheat doesn't mean you should have to sacrifice those wonderful baking smells, too.

Bread and many other baked goods get their texture, in part, from gluten. Baking without gluten yields a slightly different result. But never fear. In this chapter, we show you how delicious gluten-free baking can be. And because gluten-free baking can be a bit trickier than regular baking, we give you several tips and techniques to make it easier.

In This Chapter

- Tips for baking the perfect loaf
- Great gluten-free breads
- Crave-worthy crackers, muffins, scones, and more

Baking Tips

Baking is the cooking technique where you might miss gluten the most. You probably won't miss it when biting into a juicy rib eye or enjoying a luscious salad, but baking is a bit different.

One of the first things you might notice is that yeast breads don't rise as high or as quickly as glutenous breads. To improve their rise, preheat your oven to 200°F and then turn it off. Set a large, flat pan—like a 9×13 baking pan—full of hot water on the bottom of your oven. Pour your bread dough into the loaf pan, cover it with a damp towel, and set the bread pan in the oven on the top rack. Close the door, and let the dough rise for at least 30 minutes, or until it reaches the top of the loaf pan. When you're ready to bake, leave the pan with the water in the bottom of the oven, and preheat your oven according to your recipe. The water will create steam as the bread bakes and helps form a nice crust on the bread.

Because you have to take a few extra steps to get your gluten-free bread to rise, don't punch down the dough as you might have done with gluten-filled breads. Also, only fill your loaf pans two-thirds full. If you overfill, the dough might collapse during the baking process.

Good baking is all about precise chemistry, so measure your flours carefully. Pour the flour into a measuring cup held over a separate bowl or the sink. When the cup is completely filled, use a knife to level off the flour.

 TASTY TIDBIT

Most professional bakers don't use measurement cups but instead measure flour on scales for a more accurate reading. You don't have to do this, but you do have to be sure you measure correctly.

Also be sure your flours are at room temperature before you add the yeast. If you store your flours in the refrigerator or freezer, remove and measure the amount you need at least 1 hour before you plan to make your bread. Bring your eggs and milk to room temperature, too.

Gluten-free flours need more liquid than wheat-based flours, so when you convert nongluten recipes to gluten free, plan to add more liquid. Start by adding 1 or 2 tablespoons extra liquid. You can add more if the dough is too sticky.

Also, xanthan gum or guar gum helps ensure your bread holds together and doesn't turn into a crumbly or gooey mess.

You might like to use a digital thermometer instead of guessing when your bread is finished baking. When the internal temperature reaches 206°F, the bread is done, not dried out, and not gooey.

When you adapt recipes, note the changes and substitutions you make, so you'll remember what you did if it works. And if it doesn't work, keep a sense of humor and remember baking disasters happen even when the flour is glutenous.

You also might want to note which gluten-free flour blends you use. Most flour blends combine rice and other flours with different starches (like potato or tapioca). Jeanette uses different blends, depending on what's on sale and where she's shopping. At Trader Joe's, for example, she picks up the Trader Joe's mix. Some people swear by Bob's Red Mill; others prefer Tom Sawyer, Pamela's, Hodgson Mill, or King Arthur's.

If you're trying to decide on a brand, pick a simple baking recipe you like and make that recipe with several different brands of flour. Note the subtle (or not-so-subtle) differences among brands and what you like or don't like about certain flours so you can make a better determination.

FOOD FOR THOUGHT

If you're vegan, you can make many of the recipes in this chapter free of animal products by opting for almond milk instead of cow's milk and egg replacer instead of real eggs. Feel free to experiment to see what you like best—as long as it's gluten free.

All-Purpose Gluten-Free Flour Blend

Use this basic flour blend for making breads, muffins, and even cakes.

Yield:	Prep time:	Serving size:		
4 cups	5 minutes	2 tablespoons		
Each serving has:				
52 calories	0.2g fat	0g saturated fat	0mg cholesterol	0mg sodium
0g sugar	12g carbohydrates	0.6g fiber	0.8g protein	

1¼ cups white rice flour

1 cup brown rice flour

³/₄ cup tapioca starch

½ cup potato starch

½ cup sorghum flour

1. In a large bowl, combine white rice flour, brown rice flour, tapioca starch, potato starch, and sorghum flour.

2. Use in your favorite recipe, or store in an airtight container.

Variation: If you want to include xanthan gum in this flour blend, add 1 teaspoon. For **Whole-Wheat Flour Blend,** add ¹/₄ cup buckwheat flour and reduce the white rice flour to just 1 cup.

FOOD FOR THOUGHT

We included a serving size of 2 tablespoons here, but you might need more than that amount in your recipe. If so, keep in mind that you need to adjust the nutritional information for larger amounts, too.

☉ ☻ Basic "White" Bread

This bread recipe is an adaption of the first homemade bread Elizabeth fell in love with. It's quite delicious.

Yield:	Prep time:	Cook time:	Serving size:
1 (10×5-inch) loaf (about 10 slices)	15 minutes plus 2 hours rise time	50 to 60 minutes	1 slice

Each serving has:				
156 calories	2g fat	0g saturated fat	0mg cholesterol	382mg sodium
1.9g sugar	30.2g carbohydrates	2.6g fiber	3.9g protein	

1½ cups warm (about 110°F) water	½ cup almond flour
2 TB. brown sugar	4 TB. ground flaxseeds
2 (.25-oz.) pkg. yeast (about 2 TB.)	1 TB. xanthan gum
1 cup brown rice flour	1 TB. baking powder
1 cup white rice flour	1½ tsp. baking soda
½ cup sweet rice flour	1 tsp. sea or kosher salt
½ cup tapioca flour	

1. Grease and flour a 10×5-inch loaf pan.

2. In a small bowl, whisk together warm water, brown sugar, and yeast until dissolved. Set aside for 5 minutes to get foamy.

3. In a large bowl, mix together brown rice flour, white rice flour, sweet rice flour, tapioca flour, almond flour, flaxseeds, xanthan gum, baking powder, baking soda, and sea salt.

4. Pour yeast water over dry ingredients, stir together, and then gently knead by hand. Place dough in the prepared loaf pan, smooth the top with a spatula, cover with a towel, and set in a warm place to rise for about 2 hours.

5. Preheat the oven to 375°F.

6. Bake for 50 to 60 minutes.

7. Cool in the pan for 5 to 10 minutes, turn out onto a cooling rack, and cool for 10 more minutes.

 TASTY TIDBIT

For an extra jolt of flavor, sprinkle a mixture of ½ to 1 teaspoon each salt and sugar on top of the loaf before baking. Jeanette learned this trick from Chef Mark Weber at Jill Prescott's L'Ecole de Cuisine. It's a small thing, but it really makes the difference in the flavor of your bread.

✪ Cornbread

This is a delicious, slightly sweet cornbread with just a touch of spice, thanks to the Cajun seasoning.

Yield:	Prep time:	Cook time:	Serving size:
1 (9½×9½-inch) loaf	5 minutes	30 to 40 minutes	1 slice

Each serving has:				
141 calories	7.6g fat	4g saturated fat	46mg cholesterol	188mg sodium
1.6g sugar	16g carbohydrates	1.4g fiber	3.2g protein	

1½ cups cornmeal

1 cup corn flour

½ cup potato starch

2 TB. brown sugar

1 TB. baking powder

1 tsp. sea salt

1 tsp. xanthan gum

½ tsp. gluten-free Cajun seasoning

1¼ cups whole or 2 percent milk

½ cup melted unsalted butter

3 large eggs

1 cup frozen corn kernels, thawed

1. Preheat the oven to 350°F. Grease a 9½×9½-inch baking pan.

2. In a large bowl, combine cornmeal, corn flour, potato starch, brown sugar, baking powder, sea salt, xanthan gum, and Cajun seasoning.

3. Whisk in whole milk, butter, and eggs, and stir in corn. Pour batter into the prepared baking pan.

4. Bake for 30 to 40 minutes or until browned slightly on top and cornbread has pulled away from the edges of the pan. Slice and serve.

 TASTY TIDBIT

If you don't have any corn flour on hand, you can add 1½ cups more cornmeal instead.

⊕ ✇ Basic Pizza Crust

This is a simple and easy pizza crust to make and freeze so you can whip up pizza in a flash later.

Yield:	Prep time:	Cook time:	Serving size:
2 pizza doughs (each 8 servings)	15 minutes plus 2 hours rise time	25 to 30 minutes	1 slice

Each serving has:				
87 calories	4.9g fat	0.6g saturated fat	0mg cholesterol	145mg sodium
0.9g sugar	9.1g carbohydrates	2.3g fiber	1.9g protein	

1½ cups warm (110°F) water

1 TB. brown sugar

1 (.25-oz.) pkg. yeast (about 1 TB.)

1½ cups All-Purpose Gluten-Free Flour Blend (recipe earlier in this chapter)

½ cup cornmeal

½ cup corn flour

⅓ cup almond flour

⅓ cup ground flaxseeds

1 TB. xanthan gum

1 tsp. sea salt

1 tsp. gluten-free Italian seasoning blend

¼ cup extra-virgin olive oil

1. In a small bowl, whisk together warm water, brown sugar, and yeast until dissolved. Set aside for 5 minutes to get foamy.

2. In a large bowl, sift together All-Purpose Gluten-Free Flour Blend, cornmeal, corn flour, almond flour, flaxseeds, xanthan gum, sea salt, and Italian seasoning blend.

3. Pour yeast and water mixture over flours, and stir with a wooden spoon. Pour in olive oil, and knead gently with hands until all ingredients are incorporated. If dough is a little dry, add a bit more water, 1 tablespoon at a time, until desired consistency. Cover and let rest in a warm place for about 2 or 3 hours or until dough rises.

4. If using immediately, preheat the oven to 425°F. Lightly flour a round baking sheet with cornmeal. Divide dough into two portions, and roll one portion onto the baking sheet to ⅛ inch thickness, or about 12 to 14 inches in diameter. Add your favorite sauce and toppings, and bake for 8 to 10 minutes.

   If not using immediately, wrap tightly in plastic wrap, and refrigerate for up to 1 week or freeze for up to 1 month.

TASTY TIDBIT

If you don't have corn flour, you can use cornmeal in its place.

✸ ✿ Chickpea Flatbread

If you used to be a fan of garlic naan in Indian restaurants, you'll like this flatbread. The texture isn't exactly the same, but this flatbread boasts a delicious garlic flavor and it goes great with both Indian and Middle Eastern cuisines.

Yield:	Prep time:	Cook time:	Serving size:	
8 slices	5 minutes	8 minutes	1 slice	

Each serving has:				
122 calories	5g fat	0.7g saturated fat	0mg cholesterol	124mg sodium
3g sugar	15g carbohydrates	2.4g fiber	5g protein	

1 cup chickpea or garbanzo bean flour	$^1/_2$ tsp. onion powder
1 cup water	$^1/_2$ tsp. garlic powder
2 TB. extra-virgin olive oil	$^1/_2$ tsp. sea salt

1. Preheat the oven to 500°F. Position the oven rack about 6 inches away from the broiler. Place an ovenproof iron skillet in the oven to preheat for about 5 minutes.

2. In a medium bowl, whisk together chickpea flour, water, 1 tablespoon extra-virgin olive oil, onion powder, garlic powder, and sea salt.

3. When skillet is hot, remove from the oven, and coat the bottom with remaining 1 tablespoon extra-virgin olive oil. Pour batter into the prepared skillet, and swirl to coat evenly.

4. Bake for 5 minutes, turn on the broiler, and broil for 3 minutes or until charred slightly. Cut flatbread into 8 wedges, and serve.

Variation: For **Herbed Chickpea Flatbread,** add fresh herbs like rosemary, sage, thyme, or dill by the teaspoon. For **Olive Rosemary Flatbread,** add 1 tablespoon fresh or 1 teaspoon dried rosemary and 1 or 2 tablespoons chopped kalamata olives.

FOOD FOR THOUGHT

Enjoy this flatbread with dips, with soups, and as a bread to sop up sauces.

◉ ✪ Gluten-Free Crackers

Slightly nutty, slightly sweet, crunchy, yet delicate, these crackers make a great snack. They're also perfect for appetizers.

Yield:	Prep time:	Cook time:	Serving size:
40 crackers	30 minutes	15 minutes	2 crackers

Each serving has:				
72 calories	5.1g fat	2.6g saturated fat	0mg cholesterol	96mg sodium
0.6g sugar	4.4g carbohydrates	2.1g fiber	2g protein	

1 1/2 cups almond flour	1 tsp. baking powder
1/2 cup ground flaxseeds	1 tsp. sea salt
1/3 cup buckwheat flour	1/2 tsp. xanthan gum
1/3 cup brown rice flour	1/4 cup melted coconut oil
1 TB. brown sugar	4 TB. water

1. Preheat the oven to 300°F. Lightly grease 2 baking sheets.

2. In a large bowl, sift together almond flour, flaxseeds, buckwheat flour, brown rice flour, brown sugar, baking powder, sea salt, and xanthan gum.

3. Stir in coconut oil and water, and gently mix by hand to combine.

4. Place one small portion of dough between two silicone baking sheets or pieces of parchment paper that have been lightly brushed with oil. Use a rolling pin to roll out dough to 1/8-inch thickness, and cut out crackers using a 2 1/2-inch diameter cookie cutter that's been dipped in oil. Use a spatula to lift crackers off the silicone sheet and onto the prepared baking sheets.

5. Bake for 15 minutes. Switch baking sheets from the top rack to the bottom rack and vice versa, and bake for 15 more minutes. Remove from the oven, cool on baking sheets for 5 minutes, and transfer to cooling racks to cool completely.

Variation: If you have a dehydrator, you can dehydrate the crackers instead of baking them. Set your dehydrator for 145°F and dehydrate for 6 to 8 hours.

 FOOD FOR THOUGHT

These crackers are great to use in place of any appetizer recipes that call for little slices of pumpernickel bread. They'll also complement any recipes that go with rye bread.

❽ Banana Bread

This sweet—but not too sweet—banana bread is Jeanette's gluten-free version of her son's favorite treat.

Yield:	Prep time:	Cook time:	Serving size:
1 (10×5-inch) loaf (8 slices)	10 minutes	60 minutes	1 slice

Each serving has:				
318 calories	21g fat	12g saturated fat	41mg cholesterol	242mg sodium
22g sugar	28g carbohydrates	6g fiber	6g protein	

2 ripe bananas, peeled and mashed	¹/₂ cup ground flaxseeds
¹/₄ cup coconut oil	¹/₂ cup pecans, crushed
¹/₂ cup honey	¹/₂ cup unsweetened dried coconut flakes
¹/₂ cup coconut milk	1 TB. baking powder
2 large eggs	1 tsp. baking soda
1 tsp. vanilla extract	¹/₂ tsp. xanthan gum
1¹/₂ cups gluten-free flour	¹/₄ tsp. sea salt

1. Preheat the oven to 350°F. Grease and flour a 10×5-inch bread pan.

2. In a large bowl, and using an electric mixer on medium speed, blend bananas, coconut oil, honey, coconut milk, eggs, and vanilla extract.

3. In a separate large bowl, stir together flour, flaxseeds, pecans, coconut flakes, baking powder, baking soda, xanthan gum, and sea salt.

4. Pour dry mix into wet ingredients ¹/₂ cup at a time, and mix until well combined. Pour batter into the prepared bread pan, and bake for 60 minutes.

Variation: For a sweet **Chocolate Rum Banana Bread,** add 1 cup chocolate chips and 2 tablespoons rum.

FOOD FOR THOUGHT

Worried about serving Chocolate Rum Banana Bread to kids or those abstaining from alcohol? Replace the rum with rum extract if you like. Or you can omit the rum entirely for a tasty chocolate-only version.

☻ Pumpkin Bread

This light and sweet pumpkin bread contains just a touch of cinnamon and ginger and tastes of the flavors of autumn.

Yield:	Prep time:	Cook time:	Serving size:
1 (10×5-inch) loaf	10 minutes	60 minutes	1 slice

Each serving has:				
222 calories	1.8g fat	0.7g saturated fat	47mg cholesterol	110mg sodium
27g sugar	48g carbohydrates	3.6g fiber	3.9g protein	

1 cup fresh puréed roasted pumpkin
   or canned pumpkin

¹/₂ cup low-fat buttermilk

2 extra-large eggs

1 tsp. vanilla extract

2 cups All-Purpose Gluten-Free Flour
Blend (recipe in Chapter 18)

1 cup sugar

1 tsp. xanthan gum

1 tsp. cinnamon

¹/₂ tsp. ground ginger

1. Preheat the oven to 350°F. Lightly grease a 10×5-inch bread pan.

2. In a large bowl, whisk together puréed roasted pumpkin, buttermilk, eggs, and vanilla extract until smooth.

3. Sift All-Purpose Gluten-Free Flour Blend, sugar, xanthan gum, cinnamon, and ginger into wet ingredients, and blend until smooth.

4. Pour batter into the prepared pan. Bake for 60 minutes or until lightly browned on top.

5. Serve warm with a dollop of whipped cream or a sprinkle of confectioners' sugar and cinnamon on top.

Variation: For **Chocolate-Chip Pumpkin Bread,** add 1 cup chocolate chips to the batter after you add the dry ingredients.

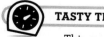

TASTY TIDBIT

This recipe really benefits from the use of a good-quality vanilla extract like Madagascar.

✪ Cranberry Orange Muffins

These muffins just shine with citrusy sweetness, and the cranberries add an extra pop of fruity flavor.

Yield:	Prep time:	Cook time:	Serving size:	
12 muffins	10 minutes	20 minutes	1 muffin	

Each serving has:				
205 calories	10g fat	0.8g saturated fat	0mg cholesterol	217mg sodium
17.7g sugar	27g carbohydrates	0g fiber	1.2g protein	

₁/₂ cup canola oil

1 cup sugar

¹/₃ cup fresh squeezed orange juice

1 TB. orange zest or zest from 1 large orange

2 large eggs

2 tsp. vanilla extract

1 cup almond flour

1 cup gluten-free flour

2 tsp. baking powder

2 tsp. baking soda

1 tsp. xanthan gum

1. Preheat the oven to 350°F. Line a 12-cup muffin pan with paper liners.

2. In a large bowl, whisk together canola oil, sugar, orange juice, orange zest, eggs, and vanilla extract.

3. Add almond flour, flour, baking powder, baking soda, and xanthan gum, and mix well. Pour batter by the ¹/₂ cupful into each muffin cup.

4. Bake for 20 minutes. Cool for 5 minutes, or serve warm from the oven.

Variation: For a kick of sweet spice, add ¹/₂ teaspoon cinnamon and/or ¹/₂ teaspoon cardamom. For a boost of fiber, add 2 tablespoons ground flaxseeds.

TASTY TIDBIT

These muffins make a great grab-and-go breakfast. Whip up a batch over the weekend, and you'll have a tasty breakfast treat for those hurried weekday mornings.

⊗ Lemon Poppy Seed Scones

Light, sweet, and just slightly tart, these scones are perfect for breakfast. They're great for afternoon tea, too.

Yield:	Prep time:	Cook time:	Serving size:
8 scones	10 minutes	20 minutes	1 scone

Each serving has:				
117 calories	6g fat	3.8g saturated fat	36mg cholesterol	117mg sodium
13g sugar	15g carbohydrates	less than 1g fiber	1.3g protein	

2¹/₂ cups gluten-free flour

¹/₂ cup sugar

5 tsp. baking powder

¹/₄ tsp. sea salt

¹/₄ tsp. xanthan gum

4 TB. unsalted butter or coconut oil

¹/₂ cup nonfat milk

1 large egg

Zest of 1 medium lemon (1 TB.)

1 TB. fresh squeezed lemon juice

1 tsp. vanilla extract

1 tsp. poppy seeds

1. Preheat the oven to 425°F.

2. In a large bowl, combine flour, sugar, baking powder, sea salt, and xanthan gum.

3. Using an electric mixer on medium speed, blend butter into dry ingredients until it looks like a crumbly mix.

4. Add milk, egg, lemon zest, lemon juice, vanilla extract, and poppy seeds, and stir until well combined.

5. On a lightly floured surface, flatten and shape dough into a 10-inch circle. Smooth it out, and use a pizza cutter to slice 8 even triangles.

6. Place triangles on a nonstick cookie sheet, and bake for 15 to 20 minutes or until lightly browned on top. Cool for 5 minutes, and serve.

Variation: For **Almond Scones,** replace the lemon juice, lemon zest, and poppy seeds with ¹/₄ cup sliced or slivered almonds and ¹/₂ teaspoons almond extract. For **Cranberry Orange Scones,** replace the lemon juice and lemon zest with orange juice and orange zest and add ¹/₂ cup dried cranberries instead of the poppy seeds. For plain **Simple Scones,** leave out the lemon juice, lemon zest, and poppy seeds.

✖ Chocolate Zucchini Bread

Even if you don't like zucchini, chances are you'll like this sweet bread that's a great way to increase your veggie intake. The chocolate chips and cocoa powder make it even more appealing.

Yield:	Prep time:	Cook time:	Serving size:
1 (5×10-inch) loaf	2 minutes	35 to 45 minutes	1 slice

Each serving has:			
480 calories	23g fat	12.8g saturated fat	77mg cholesterol 407mg sodium
38.5g sugar	64g carbohydrates	6g fiber	8g protein

2 cups gluten-free flour

$^1/_2$ cup almond flour or almond meal

1 cup sugar

$^1/_3$ cup cocoa powder

$^1/_2$ tsp. cinnamon

1 tsp. baking powder

$^1/_2$ tsp. baking soda

$^1/_2$ tsp. sea salt

$^1/_4$ tsp. xanthan gum

2 medium zucchini, shredded ($2^1/_2$ cups)

$^1/_2$ cup melted unsalted butter or vegetable oil

$^1/_2$ cup buttermilk

2 large eggs, lightly beaten

1 tsp. vanilla extract

1 cup chocolate chips

1. Preheat the oven to 350°F. Grease and flour a 5×10-inch loaf pan.

2. In a large bowl, combine flour, almond flour, sugar, cocoa powder, cinnamon, baking powder, baking soda, sea salt, and xanthan gum.

3. Stir in zucchini, butter, buttermilk, eggs, and vanilla extract. Stir in chocolate chips.

4. Pour batter into the prepared pan, and bake for 35 to 45 minutes or until top crust is hard and dough doesn't jiggle.

Variation: If you like cinnamon, increase it to 1 teaspoon.

 FOOD FOR THOUGHT

This quick bread is so delicious and chocolaty, Jeanette's husband ate the entire loaf, right out of the pan, in just one sitting. In addition, this is the only way our editor's mother has ever been able to get her to try zucchini.

CHAPTER 19

Delectable Desserts

One of the biggest challenges when eating gluten free is finding baked goods and sweets you can eat. Bakeries are often loaded with gluten, and if you're determined to stay away from it, you might be thinking you'll miss your favorite sweet treats. Not so! In this chapter, we give you recipes for great-tasting cookies, cakes, and other desserts. They're so sweet and rich, you won't miss the gluten!

We also share some baking secrets, techniques, helpful equipment, and quality ingredients you'll want to check out to create delicious desserts.

In This Chapter

- Pointers for perfect gluten-free desserts
- Better-quality ingredients yield better-tasting desserts
- Cookies, cakes, and more sweet treats

The Secret to Crumble-Free Treats

One common complaint we hear—and we have lamented ourselves—when baking gluten-free items is keeping cookies, cakes, and muffins from crumbling. Without the right binding ingredients, your gluten-free baked goods will crumble, more than any glutenous products ever did.

To prevent this, include xanthan gum and/or guar gum in your recipe. Even if your gluten-free flour blend has added xanthan gum and/or guar gum, you'll still need to add more. While testing the recipes in this chapter, for example, we needed extra binding ingredients for all different flour blends, even if the blends already contained them. When Jeanette adapts a glutenous recipe to be gluten free, she typically adds $^1/_4$ to $^1/_2$ teaspoon xanthan gum or guar gum per 1 cup gluten-free flour.

 TASTY TIDBIT

Even if your gluten-free flour mix contains guar gum or xanthan gum, add the amount called for in the recipe. It won't ruin the texture, and without it, your muffins, cakes, or cookies will definitely fall apart.

So what do you do if you added more guar gum or xanthan gum and your cookie crumbles anyway? First, look at the amount of xanthan gum or guar gum and liquid in the recipe. To correct the crumbling, start by doubling the amount of xanthan gum. If it's $^1/_2$ teaspoon, make it a full 1 teaspoon. Then, try reducing the liquid by $^1/_4$ or $^1/_2$ cup to thicken the batter. Sometimes, you need to double the xanthan gum and also reduce the liquid by 50 percent. This is also a good rule to follow when you're eliminating the gluten from a favorite glutenous dessert recipe.

You can use xanthan gum and guar gum pretty much interchangeably, but know that guar gum can clump in wet ingredients. Most gluten-free bakers have a preference for one or the other. Some aficionados experiment to find the perfect fat-flour-liquid ratio to avoid using thickening agents all together. Other bakers add $1^1/_2$ teaspoons chia seeds and $1^1/_2$ teaspoons ground flaxseeds plus 1 tablespoon boiling water and skip the xanthan gum or guar gum.

Sometimes, the simple act of freezing keeps baked goods from crumbling. So freeze your bars, cakes, or cookies after baking, and thaw them before serving. Our Gluten-Free Palmer House Brownies recipe in this chapter requires this—and it required it before we removed the gluten, too.

Better Ingredients

After flour and sugar, the most important ingredient in a baked dessert is the flavor enhancer—that is, the vanilla extract. But not all vanilla extracts are created equal. They're not equal in quality, and some vanilla extracts aren't even made from vanilla beans. Vanillin, for example, is an artificial vanilla flavoring. No vanilla beans are in the ingredients.

What's more, some vanilla extracts have a glutenous base, so use only certified gluten-free vanilla extracts. We recommend Nielsen-Massey's (nielsenmassey.com) extracts—vanilla, almond, and chocolate. All are certified gluten-free, and you can find them in many stores across the United States and Canada. Jeanette also recommends the vanilla extracts from The Spice House (thespicehouse.com) and Penzeys (penzeys.com).

Each of these companies sells different kinds and blends of vanilla extracts. Different types of vanilla offer different nuances and flavors, so it's fun to experiment with a variety of extracts. For example, Madagascar, Mexican, and Tahitian—three different types of vanilla—all have unique flavor notes. Tahitian vanilla is very delicate and floral, perfect for fruit salads and fruit desserts. Madagascar is sweeter and creamy, perfect for most baked goods. Mexican is a bit spicier and goes great with chocolate.

For an extra *oomph* of vanilla flavor, you can scrape out vanilla beans or use a vanilla bean paste. Vanilla bean paste is basically a mixture of vanilla extract, scraped beans, and sugar in paste form. If you try it, use the same amount of paste as you would extract. Nielsen-Massey makes a great paste.

 TASTY TIDBIT

To make the best desserts, always use good-quality vanilla, cream, butter, and chocolate. You really can taste the difference.

When a recipe calls for heavy cream, use only *pure* cream—heavy whipping cream with 40 percent milk fat. If it's not pure and contains creams with additives like guar gum or carrageenan, the milk fat will be lower—38 or 36 percent. Cream with additives means a mixture of cream and milk, which will break down when it's cooked or after it's whipped. Organic Valley makes a pure cream, and so does Dean's.

A Good Approach to Gluten-Free Desserts

Jeanette's philosophy for gluten-free desserts is simple: the desserts should be so good you don't miss the gluten. This sometimes requires spending a little more time in the kitchen. Our French Buttercream Frosting, for example, requires several steps, but it's so good, you'll never, ever want to get frosting out of a can or a box again. When you top your cakes with it, your family and friends will absolutely swoon.

As you become more adventurous and begin to develop your own recipes or adapt old favorites, focus first on desserts—cakes and cookies, especially—that use little flour. Soufflés, flourless chocolate cakes, and mousses and puddings are all great dishes to try. If you need a crust, crush gluten-free cookies, add some melted butter, press into a pan, and chill. It's that easy. (Be sure to check out our Flourless Chocolate Cake and Crustless Cheesecake recipes later in this chapter.)

But don't be afraid to fail. Baking is the culinary arena most prone to failure, even for experienced and educated chefs, whether gluten free or not. Learn from your missteps. Figure out what went wrong, learn from it, and make your next attempt that much better.

In fact, if your cake or muffins turn out crumbly, transform them into a tasty bread pudding. Crumble the "failed" cake or muffins into a pan, mix together 3 or 4 whisked eggs, 1 or 2 cups milk or cream, and $^1/_2$ cup sugar. Pour the egg mixture over the crumbles, and bake at 350°F for 20 to 30 minutes. You also can crumble muffins and less-sweet cakes into stuffing for a sweet/savory flavor.

FOOD FOR THOUGHT

Silicon baking sheets are a good item to have in your kitchen arsenal when baking cookies. With them, you don't have to worry about the cookies sticking to the sheets or trays. They're a good investment and last a long time.

☻ Chocolate-Chip Cookies

Perfectly chewy with a deep chocolate flavor, these cookies will become the favorite recipe of the cookie monsters in your life.

Yield:	Prep time:	Cook time:	Serving size:
24 cookies	10 minutes	12 minutes	1 cookie

Each serving has:			
206 calories	11.6g fat	5g saturated fat	28mg cholesterol 145mg sodium
11g sugar	22g carbohydrates	2.3g fiber	3.7g protein

$^3/_4$ cup brown sugar, firmly packed

$^1/_2$ cup unsalted butter (1 stick), softened

2 large eggs

1 TB. rum

1 tsp. vanilla extract

1 cup almond flour

1 cup All-Purpose Gluten-Free Flour Blend (recipe in Chapter 18)

$1^1/_2$ tsp. xanthan gum

1 tsp. baking soda

$^1/_8$ tsp. sea salt

1 cup crushed walnuts or pecans

1 (10-oz.) pkg. dark chocolate chips

1. Preheat the oven to 325°F.

2. In a large bowl, combine brown sugar and butter. Add eggs, rum, and vanilla extract, and whisk until well combined.

3. In a separate large bowl, sift together almond flour, All-Purpose Gluten-Free Flour Blend, xanthan gum, baking soda, and sea salt.

4. Whisk dry ingredients, $^1/_2$ cup at a time, into wet ingredients until well combined.

5. Stir in walnuts and dark chocolate chips.

6. Using a melon baller or teaspoon, scoop out batter onto 2 nonstick baking sheets or 2 regular sheets lined with silicon baking sheets. Using your fingers, flatten cookies and sprinkle a few grains of sea salt on each.

7. Bake for 10 to 12 minutes. Cool on a cooling rack for 5 minutes.

 TASTY TIDBIT

If you're allergic to nuts, substitute more All-Purpose Gluten-Free Flour Blend for the almond flour and leave out the walnuts. If you don't want to use rum, you can substitute with another liquor like amaretto or whiskey or just use water.

☻ Chocolate-Chunk Cookies

These ultra-thin, melt-in-your-mouth, buttery chocolate chip cookies are a favorite of guests at Napa Valley, California's Inn on Randolph.

Yield:	Prep time:	Cook time:	Serving size:
40 cookies	15 minutes	30 minutes	1 cookie

Each serving has:				
124 calories	8.7g fat	5.6g saturated fat	24mg cholesterol	120mg sodium
10.9g sugar	11.4g carbohydrates	0g fiber	.7g protein	

$1^1/_2$ cups butter (3 sticks)	2 tsp. baking soda
$2^1/_4$ cups dark brown sugar, firmly packed	$^3/_4$ tsp. xanthan gum
1 large egg	$^1/_2$ cup dark, semisweet, or milk chocolate chips, preferably large chunks
1 tsp. vanilla extract	
$2^1/_2$ cups All-Purpose Gluten-Free Flour Blend	$^1/_2$ cup white chocolate chips, preferably large chunks

1. Preheat the oven to 350°F.

2. In a large bowl, and using an electric mixer on medium speed, cream together butter and dark brown sugar.

3. Add egg and vanilla extract, and mix until well blended.

4. Add All-Purpose Gluten-Free Flour Blend, baking soda, and xanthan gum, and mix again until well blended.

5. Stir in dark chocolate chips and white chocolate chips by hand until well distributed.

6. Using a melon baller or large spoon, scoop batter onto an ungreased, nonstick baking sheet—about $1^1/_2$ tablespoons per cookie. Space cookies well apart, and only place 9 cookies per baking sheet. (Batter contains so much butter, these cookies melt and spread out quite a bit.) Lightly press down on each cookie.

7. Bake for 10 to 12 minutes. The longer you bake them, the crispier they'll be; the shorter you bake them, the chewier they'll be.

8. Remove cookies from the oven, cool on the baking sheet for 1 or 2 minutes, and transfer to a wire rack to completely cool (about 15 minutes).

Variation: For more-chocolaty cookies, add up to 1 cup more chocolate chunks of your choice.

TASTY TIDBIT

Cinnamon and chocolate go together like peanut butter and jelly. For an interesting accent, add $^1/_2$ to 1 teaspoon ground cinnamon to the batter when you mix in the All-Purpose Gluten-Free Flour Blend. The cinnamon just adds a slight, cinnamony taste—it's more of an accent to the chocolate.

❽ Oatmeal Cookies

Crunchy yet delicate, these oatmeal cookies are enhanced by coconut and cashews.

Yield:	Prep time:	Cook time:	Serving size:	
24 cookies	15 minutes	10 minutes	1 cookie	

Each serving has:				
97 calories	5.8g fat	3.8g saturated fat	0mg cholesterol	72mg sodium
7g sugar	6g carbohydrates	1.1g fiber	1.4g protein	

$1^1/_2$ cups gluten-free rolled oats

$^1/_2$ cup unsweetened shredded coconut

$^1/_2$ cup crushed cashews

2 TB. ground flaxseeds

$^1/_2$ cup honey

$^1/_4$ cup coconut oil

1 tsp. vanilla extract

1 tsp. baking soda

1 tsp. baking powder

$^1/_4$ tsp. xanthan gum

1. Preheat the oven to 350°F.

2. In a large bowl, whisk together rolled oats, coconut, cashews, flaxseeds, honey, coconut oil, vanilla extract, baking soda, baking powder, and xanthan gum.

3. Drop 2-tablespoon cookies onto a nonstick baking sheet or one lined with a silicon sheet. Using your fingers, lightly flatten each cookie.

4. Bake for 10 minutes. Cool on a cooling rack for 10 minutes.

Variation: For a little something extra, add $^1/_2$ cup dried cranberries, raisins, or chocolate chips.

 FOOD FOR THOUGHT

Normally, we use dried, unsalted nuts in recipes, but we've found that roasted, salted cashews are great to use in this recipe.

✪ Gluten-Free Palmer House Brownies

These divine brownies are extra chocolaty, chewy, and nutty.

Yield:	Prep time:	Cook time:	Serving size:
15 brownies	15 minutes	50 minutes	1 brownie

Each serving has:				
355 calories	26g fat	12g saturated fat	74mg cholesterol	119mg sodium
22g sugar	26g carbohydrates	21.6g fiber	6g protein	

1 (10-oz.) pkg. chocolate chips

1 cup unsalted butter (2 sticks), cut into chunks

$^3/_4$ cup sugar

$^1/_2$ cup All-Purpose Gluten-Free Flour Blend (recipe in Chapter 17)

$^1/_4$ cup almond flour

$1^1/_2$ tsp. baking powder

$^1/_2$ tsp. xanthan gum

3 large eggs, lightly beaten

$1^1/_2$ cups chopped walnuts or pecans

$^1/_4$ cup apricot preserves

$^1/_4$ cup plus 2 tsp. water

$^1/_8$ tsp. guar gum

1. Preheat the oven to 325°F.

2. In a large, microwave-safe bowl, melt chocolate chips and butter on high for about 2 minutes.

3. In another large bowl, whisk together sugar, All-Purpose Gluten-Free Flour Blend, almond flour, baking powder, and xanthan gum.

4. Stir in melted chocolate and butter mixture, and whisk in eggs. Batter will be thick.

5. Pour batter into an 11×7-inch baking pan, and use a spatula to smooth and even out. Sprinkle walnuts on top, and gently press them into batter.

6. Bake for about 35 to 45 minutes or until edges are slightly crisp and batter no longer jiggles in the pan. (If you stick a toothpick in it, it will test gooey.) Let cool in the pan for 20 minutes.

7. Meanwhile, in a small saucepan over medium-high heat, whisk together apricot preserves and $^1/_4$ cup water. Bring to a boil, and continue to boil for about 2 or 3 minutes.

8. In a small bowl, whisk together guar gum and remaining 2 teaspoons water. Whisk guar gum paste into apricot mixture, reduce heat to medium, and continue to whisk until guar gum paste is completely dissolved and apricot mixture is thickened.

9. When brownies have cooled, brush glaze on top. (You won't use all this glaze. Use the left-overs on meat or fish or to flavor yogurt.)

10. Cut brownies but do not remove from the pan. Place entire plan of brownies in the freezer for 3 or 4 hours. Remove, let warm to room temperature for 10 minutes, and serve.

Variation: You can omit the nuts if you have an allergy.

 FOOD FOR THOUGHT

Brownies were first invented at the Palmer House Hilton in Chicago for the Columbia Exposition. This version of the hotel's famous dessert eliminates the gluten but stays true to the original recipe's taste and texture.

🌀 Vanilla Cake with French Buttercream Frosting

This layer cake is delicious and spongy, but what's on top is absolutely decadent. The frosting, although a bit tricky to make at first, is well worth the effort.

Yield:	Prep time:	Cook time:	Serving size:
1 (9-inch) layer cake (8 slices)	15 minutes	20 to 30 minutes	1 slice

Each serving has:				
754 calories	48g fat	30g saturated fat	231mg cholesterol	372mg sodium
51g sugar	76g carbohydrates	1.1g fiber	5.3g protein	

2 cups All-Purpose Gluten-Free Flour Blend (recipe in Chapter 17)	2 tsp. vanilla extract
2 TB. baking powder	Pinch sea salt
$1/3$ tsp. xanthan gum	$1/3$ cup water
$1/2$ cup unsalted butter or vegetable oil	1 large egg white
2 cups sugar	$1/4$ tsp. cream of tartar
3 large eggs	2 large egg yolks
$3/4$ cup nonfat milk	$1 1/2$ cups unsalted butter (3 sticks), cut into 1-in. chunks

1. Preheat the oven to 375°F. Grease and flour 2 (9-inch) cake pans. Set aside.

2. In a large bowl, stir together All-Purpose Gluten-Free Flour Blend, baking powder, and xanthan gum. Set aside.

3. In another large bowl, and using an electric mixer on high speed, beat $1/2$ cup butter and 1 cup sugar until creamy.

4. Add 3 eggs and flour mixture, and beat on medium until well combined.

5. Add milk, 1 teaspoon vanilla extract and sea salt, and mix until well combined. Batter will be thick.

6. Evenly divide batter between cake pans, and bake for 20 minutes or until golden and no longer jiggly in the middle. Completely cool in the pan or on a cooling rack before frosting.

7. Meanwhile, in a medium saucepan over high heat, combine 1 cup sugar and water. Cook, stirring frequently and checking the temperature often on a candy thermometer, until temperature reaches about 230°F and starts boiling.

8. Immediately, in a medium bowl and using an electric mixer on medium speed, whip egg white and cream of tartar. Keep watching the candy thermometer. As soon as the thermometer reaches 248°F, remove from heat, and slowly pour $^1/_2$ of sugar water mixture into egg whites. Increase mixer speed to high, add egg yolks, and slowly pour in rest of sugar water mixture. When combined, reduce speed to medium, and as soon as mixture has cooled (after about 2 or 3 minutes of whipping), turn off mixer.

9. Using a spatula, remove any sugar mixture that's started to solidify on the bowl.

10. Begin adding remaining $1^1/_2$ cups butter, a chunk or two at a time, mixing on medium speed. When all butter has been added, beat on high for 2 or 3 minutes or until lustrous and creamy.

11. Add remaining 1 teaspoon vanilla extract, and beat for 1 more minute.

12. Frost cake, slice, and serve.

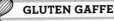 **GLUTEN GAFFE**

In theory, the heat of the syrup cooks the egg whites and yolks. In practice, it doesn't because the mixing bowl cools them. Because of concerns regarding salmonella, it's best to use pasteurized eggs, or eggs that come from a local source you trust, in this recipe.

☻ Carrot Cake with Cream Cheese Frosting

Sweet, but not too sweet, this moist, rich carrot cake is a perfect summer dessert.

Yield:	Prep time:	Cook time:	Serving size:	
1 (9×13-inch) cake (20 slices)	20 minutes	30 minutes	1 slice	

Each serving has:				
211 calories	16g fat	8.7g saturated fat	70mg cholesterol	319mg sodium
12g sugar	15g carbohydrates	1.3g fiber	3.2g protein	

1 lb. carrots, peeled and grated (about 4 cups)

1 (20-oz.) can crushed pineapple, drained

1 (1-in.) piece fresh ginger, peeled

$^1/_2$ cup unsalted butter (1 stick) or coconut oil

$^3/_4$ cup brown sugar, firmly packed

$^1/_4$ cup maple syrup

4 tsp. vanilla extract

4 large eggs, lightly beaten

3 cups gluten-free flour

1 TB. baking soda

1 TB. baking powder

1 tsp. xanthan gum

1 tsp. cinnamon

$^1/_2$ tsp. nutmeg

$^1/_2$ cup chopped walnuts or pecans

$^1/_2$ cup unsalted butter (1 stick)

1 (8-oz.) pkg. low-fat cream cheese

1 cup confectioners' sugar

1 or 2 TB. milk (optional)

1. Preheat the oven to 350°F. Grease and flour a 9×13-inch cake pan.

2. In a food processor fitted with a standard blade, purée carrots, pineapple, and ginger.

3. In a large bowl, and using an electric mixer on medium speed, whip together $^1/_2$ cup butter, brown sugar, maple syrup, and 2 teaspoons vanilla extract for 3 minutes.

4. Add eggs, and beat for 5 minutes or until well combined.

5. Add puréed carrot mixture, and stir by hand until combined.

6. In another large bowl, sift together flour, baking soda, baking powder, xanthan gum, cinnamon, and nutmeg.

7. Stir dry ingredients into wet ingredients $^1/_2$ cup at a time until well combined. Stir in walnuts.

8. Pour batter into the prepared pan, and bake for 30 minutes. Let cool for 30 minutes.

9. Meanwhile, in a large bowl and using an electric mixer on medium speed, whip together remaining $1/2$ cup butter, cream cheese, confectioners' sugar, and remaining 2 teaspoons vanilla extract. Add a little milk if mixture is too thick.

10. Frost cake, slice, and serve.

Variation: For an extra touch of sweetness, you can add 1 cup raisins if you like.

FOOD FOR THOUGHT

According to the World Carrot Museum (carrotmuseum.co.uk), one of the first references to carrot cake date to 1783. In her *New York Cookbook,* Molly O'Neill writes, "George Washington was served a carrot tea cake at Fraunces Tavern in lower Manhattan" on November 25, 1783.

✪ Chocolate Cake with Chocolate Ganache

Light and almost spongy, this rich chocolate cake has a velvety texture, and the delicious chocolate ganache makes it even more decadent.

Yield:	Prep time:	Cook time:	Serving size:
1 (8-inch) cake (8 slices)	30 minutes	30 minutes	1 slice

Each serving has:				
426 calories	31g fat	19g saturated fat	121mg cholesterol	551mg sodium
24g sugar	29g carbohydrates	2.2g fiber	5.7g protein	

10 oz. bittersweet chocolate, broken into pieces

$^1/_2$ cup plus 2 TB. unsalted butter

$^1/_2$ cup plus 2 TB. sugar

Zest of 1 medium orange

2 TB. Grand Marnier

3 large eggs, separated

$^1/_3$ cup almond flour

2 TB. All-Purpose Gluten-Free Flour Blend (recipe in Chapter 17)

$^1/_4$ tsp. cream of tartar

Pinch sea salt

1 tsp. vanilla extract

$^2/_3$ cup heavy cream

1. Preheat the oven to 325°F. Place the oven rack in the lower-middle part of the oven. Grease an 8-inch cake pan. Cut an 8-inch circle of parchment paper, place in the cake pan, and grease top of parchment paper. Lightly flour sides of pan and parchment paper.

2. In a small microwave-safe bowl, melt 4 ounces bittersweet chocolate on high for 1 minute.

3. In a large bowl, and using an electric mixer on medium-low speed, cream $^1/_2$ cup butter and $^1/_2$ cup sugar for 2 minutes or until fluffy.

4. Add orange zest and Grand Marnier, and beat for 1 minute.

5. Add egg yolks, and whip for about 30 seconds or until smooth. Pour in melted chocolate, and beat for 2 or 3 minutes or until well blended and smooth.

6. In a separate large bowl, stir together almond flour and All-Purpose Gluten-Free Flour Blend. Slowly stir flours into chocolate mixture.

7. In a clean bowl, and using an electric mixer on medium speed, whip egg whites for about 2 minutes or until slightly foamy.

8. Add cream of tartar and sea salt, and whip for 3 to 5 more minutes or until soft peaks form.

9. Add remaining 2 tablespoons sugar, and whip 1 more minute or until stiff, glossy peaks form.

10. Add vanilla extract, and beat for 30 more seconds or until just combined.

11. Using a large rubber spatula, gently fold egg whites into chocolate mixture, 1 spoonful at a time. Batter will smooth, but don't overmix—you don't want to deflate egg whites.

12. Pour batter into the prepared cake pan, smoothing top with the spatula.

13. Bake for 30 minutes or until edges pull slightly away from the pan and cake no longer jiggles in the middle.

14. Cool in the pan for 30 minutes on a cooling rack. Loosen edges of cake from the pan with a knife, and gently unmold onto the cooling rack.

15. Meanwhile, in a large microwave-safe bowl, melt remaining 6 ounces bittersweet chocolate and remaining 2 tablespoons butter on high for 1 minute.

16. In a small saucepan over low heat, heat heavy cream for about 2 minutes or until just warmed.

17. Pour cream over chocolate and butter mixture, and whisk gently until smooth.

18. To frost cake, pour about $^1/_3$ of ganache on top of cake, in the center, and use a spatula to spread evenly across top and down sides of cake. Pour more ganache in the middle, as needed. Lots of ganache will drip off cake—that's okay.

19. Let cake stand for 30 minutes in cool room or the refrigerator so ganache will set. Slice and serve.

TASTY TIDBIT

The trickiest part of making this cake is folding in the egg whites without breaking them down. Here's how: put a dollop of egg whites in the middle of the batter, and cut through the egg whites, slicing in the middle to the bottom of the bowl. As you scoop the egg whites through the batter, circle your spatula, with the egg whites on it, around the edge of the bowl, and fold them gently on top of the egg whites that are still sitting on the batter. Turn the bowl a quarter, scoop, fold, and repeat. Keep adding the egg whites, folding them in gently until they are completely incorporated.

Flourless Chocolate Cake

This flour-free cake is like a large chocolate truffle. It's especially delightful served with a mound of pure whipped cream on top. Pure chocolate bliss.

Yield:	Prep time:	Cook time:	Serving size:
1 (10-inch) cake (8 slices)	5 minutes	30 minutes, plus 1 hour freeze time	1 slice

Each serving has:				
423 calories	24.6g fat	15.4g saturated fat	226mg cholesterol	668mg sodium
39g sugar	38g carbohydrates	81.9g fiber	7.5g protein	

16 oz. bittersweet chocolate, chopped or grated

2 TB. unsalted butter

7 large egg yolks plus 1 whole egg, or just 9 egg yolks

¹/₈ cup sugar

¹/₄ cup pure heavy cream

¹/₄ cup amaretto, Grand Marnier, or your favorite liquor

Toasted almond bits or mandarin orange segments

1. In a double boiler over medium-low heat, melt bittersweet chocolate and butter.

2. Add egg yolks, sugar, heavy cream, and amaretto, and stir for 2 minutes or until completely combined. Remove from heat.

3. Line a 10-inch baking pan with plastic wrap. Pour chocolate mixture into the pan, and refrigerate for 4 hours or freeze for 1 hour. (You can freeze for up to 1 week before serving.)

4. Unmold cake onto a plate, top with almonds or mandarin oranges, and serve.

 FOOD FOR THOUGHT

Using pure heavy cream is very important in this recipe. Pure cream means the ingredient list is only heavy cream—no guar gum, carrageenan, or other thickening ingredients. When the latter are added, the result isn't really pure heavy cream—it's a mixture of milk and cream. The additives break down when you heat them, which is why, you sometimes see puddles of milk when you top a slice of pie with whipped cream. Pure cream doesn't break down and is much better for baking.

Crustless Cheesecake

This is actually a rather healthy dessert, believe it or not. Best of all, it's light, fluffy, and tastes delicious.

Yield:	Prep time:	Cook time:	Serving size:
1 (12-inch) cake (10 slices)	15 minutes	30 minutes	1 slice

Each serving has:				
90 calories	2.5g fat	1.5g saturated fat	10mg cholesterol	250mg sodium
8g sugar	9g carbohydrates	0g fiber	9g protein	

6 large egg whites	2 tsp. fresh squeezed lemon juice
1 tsp. vanilla extract	4 oz. low-fat cream cheese
2 cups low-fat cottage cheese	¼ cup agave nectar
1 tsp. lemon zest	

1. Preheat the oven to 350°F. Line a 12-inch spring-form pan with aluminum foil, being sure the foil fits the pan tightly and the bottom is smooth and has no creases or folds (this will be the top of your cheesecake). Spray the foil with cooking spray.

2. In a large bowl, and using an electric mixer on high speed, beat egg whites for about 2 minutes or until soft peaks form.

3. Add vanilla extract, and beat for a few more seconds or until combined.

4. In a food processor fitted with a standard blade, purée cottage cheese, lemon zest, and lemon juice for about 3 minutes or until smooth.

5. Add cream cheese and agave nectar, and purée for about 2 more minutes or until well blended.

6. Gently fold cheese mixture into egg whites. (Some of egg whites might break down during the mixing, but that's fine.)

7. Pour batter into the prepared pan, and place the pan into another, larger pan filled with 1 inch water. Bake for 30 minutes or until cheesecake is set and slightly golden on top.

8. Remove cheesecake from water bath, and let sit for at least 5 minutes before serving.

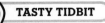 **TASTY TIDBIT**

You can make this cake several hours ahead or even overnight, and refrigerate until ready to serve with whipped cream and/or fruit topping.

Ⓥ Mango-Pineapple Coulis

This sweet and rich syrup is bursting with pineapple and mango flavor. It's wonderful served over any number of desserts, from cakes to ice cream, as well as other nondessert foods.

Yield:	Prep time:	Cook time:	Serving size:
2 cups	5 minutes, plus 1 hour cool time	10 minutes	2 tablespoons

Each serving has:				
18 calories	0g fat	0g saturated fat	0mg cholesterol	0mg sodium
4.3g sugar	4.4g carbohydrates	0g fiber	0g protein	

1 cup frozen mango chunks, thawed

1 cup frozen pineapple chunks, thawed

1 TB. agave nectar

1 tsp. vanilla extract

1. In a food processor fitted with a standard S-blade or a blender, purée mango, pineapple, agave nectar, vanilla extract for 5 minutes or until smooth.

2. Pour mixture into a medium saucepan, set over medium-low heat, and cook, stirring occasionally, for about 10 minutes or until thick.

3. Refrigerate for 1 hour before serving over Crustless Cheesecake (recipe earlier in this chapter).

DEFINITION

Coulis is fruits (or vegetables) puréed and then often headed and cooled. It's most often served as a garnish or sauce for other foods.

◍ Faux Chocolate Mousse

This tastes like whipped chocolate mousse, but the calories are much, much lower than the real thing.

Yield:	Prep time:	Cook time:	Serving size:
²/₃ cup	5 minutes	10 minutes	¹/₃ cup

Each serving has:				
288 calories	14.7g fat	10.3g saturated fat	11mg cholesterol	41mg sodium
25.8g sugar	30g carbohydrates	1.8g fiber	3.8g protein	

3.5 oz. dark chocolate, preferably
    70 percent or darker

¹/₃ cup water

1 TB. coffee liqueur

1 tsp. Mexican vanilla extract

¹/₄ tsp. cinnamon

Dash cayenne

Cocoa powder

1. In a food processor fitted with a standard S-blade, chop dark chocolate for about 3 minutes or until it's the consistency of coffee grounds.

2. Fill a large bowl with ice and water. Set a smaller bowl on top of the ice. Set aside.

3. In a small saucepan over medium heat, combine chopped chocolate, ¹/₃ cup water, coffee liqueur, Mexican vanilla extract, cinnamon, and cayenne. Cook for 2 or 3 minutes or until chocolate is melted and it's the consistency of chocolate syrup.

4. Immediately remove from heat and pour into the small bowl on top of the ice and water.

5. Use large whisk, whip chocolate sauce until it thickens into "mousse." After about 2 or 3 minutes of whisking, chocolate sauce will thicken to the consistency of instant chocolate pudding. Whisk for about 30 to 45 more seconds. When finished, it will have the consistency of chocolate mousse or nondairy whipped topping. Be careful not to overwhisk.

6. Scoop into bowls, and serve immediately. Garnish with cocoa powder or extra coffee liqueur drizzled on top.

Variation: Instead of coffee liqueur and cinnamon with a touch of heat from the cayenne pepper, you can make a sweeter **Faux Orange-Chocolate Mousse** using 1 tablespoon Grand Marnier and ¹/₄ teaspoon orange zest and omitting the cayenne.

FOOD FOR THOUGHT

This dessert works best if you use a high-quality, very dark or bittersweet chocolate, preferably 70 percent cocoa or darker. Dandelion chocolate bars (made with just cocoa beans and sugar) work well in this recipe (dandelionchocolate.com).

Gluten-Free Piecrust

This flaky, buttery crust is perfect for pies, quiches, and tarts.

Yield:	Prep time:	Cook time:	Serving size:
1 (9-inch) piecrust	1^1/$_2$ hours	20 minutes	^{1}/$_8$ pie

Each serving has:				
187 calories	19g fat	11g saturated fat	69mg cholesterol	275mg sodium
21g sugar	3g carbohydrates	0.6g fiber	1.6g protein	

^{3}/$_4$ cup All-Purpose Gluten-Free Flour Blend (recipe in Chapter 17)

^{3}/$_4$ cup almond flour

^{1}/$_2$ tsp. sea salt

^{3}/$_4$ cup unsalted butter (1^1/$_2$ sticks), very cold

1 large egg, lightly beaten

1 TB. water

1. On a clean counter or extra-large cutting board, sift together All-Purpose Gluten-Free Flour Blend, almond flour, and sea salt.

2. Chop butter into flour mixture using two knives or a pastry cutter until a rough, crumbly mixture forms.

3. Form mixture into a mound, making a small well in the center. Pour egg and water into the well, and chop with the knives or pastry cutter to incorporate.

4. Using the heel of your hand, smear dough across the clean counter until dough forms. (You only need to smear 2 or 3 times to blend well, and there will still be some tiny chunks of butter in dough.)

5. Divide dough into two balls, and flatten into discs. Wrap in plastic wrap, and refrigerate for 1 hour or up to 24 hours before using. You can also freeze dough for up to 1 month before using.

6. Preheat the oven to 400°F.

7. Place a sheet of parchment paper on the counter, and using a rolling pin, roll dough to ^{1}/$_8$ inch thick and about 10 inches in diameter. Use the parchment paper to gently transfer the dough into a 9-inch pie pan.

8. To bake without filling, pierce crust with a fork several times, line crust with parchment paper, and fill with pie weights. Bake for 10 minutes, remove pie weights, and bake 5 to 10 more minutes or until crust is lightly browned. Cool for 10 minutes before filling.

 TASTY TIDBIT

You can make the dough in a food processor, skipping the blending and the smearing process, but the crust won't be as light or flaky.

Pumpkin Pie

Fresh pumpkin, roasted before making the pie, and a little bit of rum make this one sensational pie perfect for fall and winter holidays.

Yield:	Prep time:	Cook time:	Serving size:	
1 (9-inch) pie	2 minutes	30 minutes	$^1/_8$ pie	
Each serving has:				
397 calories	27g fat	15g saturated fat	160mg cholesterol	312mg sodium
26g sugar	32g carbohydrates	1.4g fiber	5g protein	

1 Gluten-Free Piecrust, unbaked

2 cups fresh pumpkin purée from 1 small pie pumpkin

$^3/_4$ cup dark brown sugar, firmly packed

$^1/_4$ cup maple syrup

1 TB. arrowroot powder

1 tsp. cinnamon

1 tsp. pumpkin pie spice

$^1/_2$ tsp. nutmeg

3 large eggs

1 cup heavy cream

$^1/_4$ cup whole milk

$^1/_4$ cup rum

2 tsp. vanilla extract

1. Preheat the oven to 400°F.

2. Bake Gluten-Free Piecrust for 10 minutes filled with pie weights. After 10 minutes, remove crust from the oven, and reduce heat to 375°F.

3. In a large bowl, whisk together pumpkin purée, dark brown sugar, maple syrup, arrowroot powder, cinnamon, pumpkin pie spice, and nutmeg.

4. Whisk in eggs, heavy cream, milk, rum, and vanilla extract.

5. Pour filling into crust, and bake for 20 minutes. Reduce heat to 325°F, and bake for 30 more minutes or until filling no longer jiggles when shaken.

6. Cool for 20 minutes before topping with whipped cream or ice cream and serving.

Variation: You can substitute 1 (16-ounce) can pumpkin for the fresh. If you don't have pumpkin pie spice, you can use $^1/_2$ teaspoon mace, $^1/_2$ teaspoon ginger, $^1/_4$ teaspoon allspice, and $^1/_4$ teaspoon cloves. You also can eliminate the rum if you like.

TASTY TIDBIT

This recipe is exceptional if you use fresh pumpkin purée. To make, preheat the oven to 350ºF. Place a pie pumpkin on a baking sheet and bake for 60 minutes. Let cool. Cut pumpkin, remove the seeds and the skin, and purée chunks of pumpkin in a food processor fitted with a standard S-blade.

Glossary

al dente Italian for "against the teeth," this term refers to pasta or rice that's neither soft nor hard but just slightly firm against the teeth.

allspice A spice named for its flavor echoes of several spices (cinnamon, cloves, nutmeg) used in many desserts and in rich marinades and stews.

almond flour A gluten-free flour milled from skinned almonds. Almonds provide antioxidants along with potassium, magnesium, niacin, alpha-tocopherol, calcium, iron, and protein. Almond flour is great in bread and cookie recipes.

amaranth A small, yellowish seed loaded with lots of amino acids and protein.

antioxidant A substance found in foods that helps prevent the food from oxidizing or becoming rotten. Some scientists suggest that antioxidants can help reduce heart disease and cancer. Vitamins E and C are antioxidants.

antipasto A classic Italian-style appetizer that includes an assortment of meats, cheeses, and vegetables such as prosciutto, capicolla, mozzarella, mushrooms, and olives.

arborio rice A plump Italian rice used for, among other purposes, risotto.

artichoke heart The center part of the artichoke flower, often found canned in grocery stores.

arrowroot A gluten-free thickening agent made from a tropical tuber that has two times the thickening power of wheat flour. It's tasteless and clear and thickens at a lower temperature than cornstarch and wheat. Arrowroot is especially great when needing to thicken a fruit sauce or filling.

artisan Food that's hand crafted in small batches. Can also be person who hand crafts food.

arugula A spicy-peppery green with leaves that resemble a dandelion and have a distinctive and very sharp flavor.

bake To cook in a dry oven. Dry-heat cooking often results in a crisping of the exterior of the food being cooked. Moist-heat cooking, through methods such as steaming, poaching, etc., brings a much different, moist quality to the food.

baking powder A dry ingredient used to increase volume and lighten or leaven baked goods.

balsamic vinegar Vinegar produced primarily in Italy from a specific type of grape and aged in wood barrels. It's heavier, darker, and sweeter than most vinegars.

basil A flavorful, almost sweet, resinous herb delicious with tomatoes and used in all kinds of Italian- and Mediterranean-style dishes.

baste To keep foods moist during cooking by spooning, brushing, or drizzling with a liquid.

beat To quickly mix substances.

Belgian endive *See* endive.

blacken To cook something quickly in a very hot skillet over high heat, usually with a seasoning mixture.

blanch To place a food in boiling water for about 1 minute or less to partially cook the exterior and then submerge in or rinse with cool water to halt the cooking.

blend To completely mix something, usually with a blender or food processor, slower than beating.

boil To heat a liquid to the point where water is forced to turn into steam, causing the liquid to bubble. To boil something is to insert it into boiling water. A rapid boil is when a lot of bubbles form on the surface of the liquid.

bok choy A member of the cabbage family with thick stems, crisp texture, and fresh flavor. It's perfect for stir-frying.

bouillon Dried essence of stock from chicken, beef, vegetables, or other ingredients. It's a popular starting ingredient for soups because it adds flavor (and often a lot of salt).

braise To cook with the introduction of some liquid, usually over an extended period of time.

brine A highly salted, often seasoned, liquid used to flavor and preserve foods. To brine a food is to soak, or preserve, it by submerging it in brine. The salt in the brine penetrates the fibers of the meat and makes it moist and tender.

broil To cook in a dry oven under the overhead high-heat element.

broth *See* stock.

brown To cook in a skillet, turning, until the food's surface is seared and brown in color, to lock in the juices.

brown rice   A whole-grain rice, including the germ, with a characteristic pale brown or tan color. It's more nutritious and flavorful than white rice.

bruschetta (or **crostini**)   Slices of toasted or grilled bread with garlic and olive oil, often with other toppings.

buckwheat   A gluten-free seed. It can be ground into flour and offers a hearty, whole grain–like taste.

bulgur   A wheat kernel that's been steamed, dried, and crushed and is sold in fine and coarse textures.

canapé   A bite-size hors d'oeuvre usually served on a small piece of bread or toast.

caper   The flavorful buds of a Mediterranean plant, ranging in size from *nonpareil* (about the size of a small pea) to larger, grape-size caper berries produced in Spain.

caramelize   To cook sugar over low heat until it develops a sweet caramel flavor, or to cook vegetables (especially onions) or meat in butter or oil over low heat until they soften, sweeten, and develop a caramel color.

caraway   A distinctive spicy seed used for bread, pork, cheese, and cabbage dishes. It's known to reduce stomach upset, which is why it's often paired with foods like sauerkraut.

carbohydrate   A nutritional component found in starches, sugars, fruits, and vegetables that causes a rise in blood glucose levels. Carbohydrates supply energy and many important nutrients, including vitamins, minerals, and antioxidants.

cardamom   An intense, sweet-smelling spice used in baking and coffee and common in Indian cooking.

carob   A tropical tree that produces long pods from which the dried, baked, and powdered flesh—carob powder—is used in baking. The flavor is sweet and reminiscent of chocolate.

cayenne   A fiery spice made from hot chile peppers, especially the cayenne chile, a slender, red, and very hot pepper.

celiac disease   A genetic autoimmune disease that can be characterized by the destruction of villi in the small intestine and malnutrition. Its only treatment, to date, is the avoidance of gluten. Also called *celiac sprue*.

ceviche   A seafood dish in which fresh fish or seafood is marinated for several hours in highly acidic lemon or lime juice, tomato, onion, and cilantro. The acid "cooks" the seafood.

chèvre   A creamy-salty soft goat cheese. Chèvres vary in style from mild and creamy to aged, firm, and flavorful.

chickpea   A roundish yellow-gold bean used as the base ingredient in hummus. Chickpeas are high in fiber and low in fat. Also called garbanzo bean.

chickpea flour   A gluten-free flour, also called garbanzo bean flour, ground from chickpeas. Chickpea flour has higher protein content than grain flour and is good as a thickener. Use it in breads; it's also good for falafel patties and to coat foods before frying.

chile   Any one of many different "hot" peppers, ranging in intensity from the relatively mild ancho pepper to the blisteringly hot habanero.

chili powder   A warm, rich seasoning blend that includes chile pepper, cumin, garlic, and oregano.

Chinese five-spice powder   A pungent mixture of equal parts cinnamon, cloves, fennel seed, anise, and Szechuan peppercorns.

chive   A member of the onion family, chives grow in bunches of long leaves that resemble tall grass or the green tops of onions and offer a light onion flavor.

chop   To cut into pieces, usually qualified by an adverb such as "*coarsely* chopped" or by a size measurement such as "chopped into $1/2$-inch pieces." "Finely chopped" is much closer to mince.

chorizo   A spiced pork sausage often used in Mexican dishes.

chutney   A thick condiment often served with Indian curries made with fruits and/or vegetables with vinegar, sugar, and spices.

cider vinegar   A vinegar produced from apple cider, popular in North America.

cilantro   A member of the parsley family used in Mexican dishes (especially salsa) and some Asian dishes. Use in moderation because the flavor can overwhelm. The seed of the cilantro plant is the spice coriander.

cinnamon   A rich, aromatic spice commonly used in baking or desserts. Cinnamon can also be used for delicious and interesting entrées.

clove   A sweet, strong, almost wintergreen-flavor spice used in baking.

coconut flour   A gluten-free flour made from dried and defatted coconut. The flour requires using a lot more liquid than other flours; some chefs recommend using double the amount of liquid in a recipe. It's good in pancakes and waffles but also can be good in some cakes.

community supported agriculture (CSA)   A cooperative group of people to whom a farmer sells shares of or a subscription to his or her crops. At regular intervals throughout a growing season, such as once a week, the consumer picks up the fresh farm foods from a central location. Many food cooperatives and health food stores help promote CSAs.

compote　Fruit that has been cooked slowly in a simple syrup so it retains its shape and is then chilled.

coriander　A rich, warm, spicy seed used in all types of recipes, from African to South American, from entrées to desserts.

cornstarch　A thickener used in baking and food processing. It's the refined starch of the endosperm of the corn kernel. To avoid clumps, it's often mixed with cold liquid to make into a paste before adding to a recipe.

count　In terms of seafood or other foods that come in small sizes, the number of that item that compose 1 pound. For example, 31 to 40 count shrimp are large appetizer shrimp often served with cocktail sauce; 51 to 60 count are much smaller.

couscous　Granular semolina (durum wheat) that's cooked and used in many Mediterranean and North African dishes.

cream　To beat a fat such as butter, often with another ingredient such as sugar, to soften and aerate a batter.

crimini mushroom　A relative of the white button mushroom that's brown in color and has a richer flavor. The larger, fully grown version is the portobello. *See also* portobello mushroom.

crudité　Fresh vegetables served as an appetizer, often all together on one tray.

cumin　A fiery, smoky-tasting spice popular in Middle Eastern and Indian dishes. Cumin is a seed; ground cumin seed is the most common form used in cooking.

cure　To preserve uncooked foods, usually meats or fish, by either salting and smoking or pickling.

curry　Rich, spicy, Indian-style sauces and the dishes prepared with them. A curry uses curry powder as its base seasoning.

curry powder　A ground blend of rich and flavorful spices used as a basis for curry and many other Indian-influenced dishes. Common ingredients include hot pepper, nutmeg, cumin, cinnamon, pepper, and turmeric. Some curry can also be found in paste form.

custard　A cooked mixture of eggs and milk popular as a base for desserts.

dal　A dried pea, bean, or legume used in Indian cooking. Also sometimes called *urad*, *toovar*, *massor*, and *mung*.

dash　A few drops, usually of a liquid, released by a quick shake.

deglaze　To scrape up bits of meat and seasoning left in a pan or skillet after cooking. Usually this is done by adding a liquid such as wine or broth and creating a flavorful stock that can be used to create sauces.

devein To remove the dark vein from the back of a large shrimp with a sharp knife.

dice To cut into small cubes about $1/4$-inch square.

Dijon mustard A hearty, spicy mustard made in the style of the Dijon region of France.

dill A herb perfect for eggs, salmon, cheese dishes, and, of course, vegetables (pickles!).

dollop A spoonful of something creamy and thick, like sour cream or whipped cream.

double boiler A set of two pots designed to nest together, one inside the other, and provide consistent, moist heat for foods that need delicate treatment. The bottom pot holds water (not quite touching the bottom of the top pot); the top pot holds the food you want to heat.

dredge To coat a piece of food on all sides with a dry substance such as gluten-free breadcrumbs or cornmeal.

drizzle To lightly sprinkle drops of a liquid over food, often as the finishing touch to a dish.

edamame Fresh, plump, pale green soybeans, similar in appearance to lima beans, often served steamed and either shelled or still in their protective pods.

emulsion A combination of liquid ingredients that don't normally mix well (such as a fat or oil with water) that are beaten together to create a thick liquid. Creating emulsions must be done carefully and rapidly to ensure the particles of one ingredient are suspended in the other.

en papillote A French term that refers to wrapping food inside oiled parchment paper. As the food steams inside the paper, the parchment paper expands and puffs out. When serving, slit open the paper to reveal the cooked food.

endive A green that resembles a small, elongated, tightly packed head of romaine lettuce. The thick, crunchy leaves can be broken off and used with dips and spreads.

entrée The main dish in a meal.

extra-virgin olive oil *See* olive oil.

extract A concentrated flavoring derived from foods or plants through evaporation or distillation that imparts a powerful flavor without altering the volume or texture of a dish.

falafel A Middle Eastern food made of seasoned, ground chickpeas formed into balls, cooked, and often used as a filling in pitas.

fava bean flour An earthy-tasting gluten-free flour made from fava beans. Some people love using this flour in breads and pizzas.

fennel In seed form, a fragrant, licorice-tasting herb. The bulbs have a mild flavor and a celery-like crunch and are used as a vegetable in salads or cooked recipes.

flour   Grains ground into a meal. Wheat is perhaps the most common flour, but oats, rye, buckwheat, soybeans, chickpeas, etc. can also be used, as well as a variety of gluten-free flours.

fold   To combine a dense and light mixture with a circular action from the middle of the bowl.

frittata   A skillet-cooked mixture of eggs and other ingredients that's not stirred but is cooked slowly and then either flipped or finished under the broiler.

fry   *See* sauté.

garfava flour   A gluten-free made from a blend of garbanzo bean flour, or chickpea flour, and fava bean flour. This nutty-tasting flour has a high protein content and stands up well when combined with other gluten-free flours sorghum or millet.

garlic   A member of the onion family, a pungent and flavorful vegetable used in many savory dishes. A garlic bulb contains multiple cloves. Each clove, when chopped, provides about 1 teaspoon garlic.

ginger   A flavorful root available fresh or dried and ground that adds a pungent, sweet, and spicy quality to a dish.

gluten   A protein found in wheat and other cereal grains. Throughout the book we use the term *gluten* to refer to the element in wheat, barley, rye, and wheat's relatives that consistently proves to be problematic for those suffering from gluten intolerance.

glutened   The act of eating gluten when either you've been told there's no gluten in a dish or when you eat hidden gluten and feel ill afterward.

Greek yogurt   A strained yogurt that's a good natural source of protein, calcium, and probiotics. Greek yogurt averages 40 percent more protein per ounce than traditional yogurt.

groats   Hulled cereal grains, such as oats, wheat, barley, and rye, as well as hulled grainlike seeds such as buckwheat. Groats are whole grains and are often used in soups and porridges.

guar gum   A gluten-free thickening agent made from a plant in the legume family.

handful   An unscientific measurement, it's the amount of an ingredient you can hold in your hand.

hazelnut flour   A gluten-free flour made from hazelnuts. Use to enrich the taste and texture of baked goods, especially cakes and cookies.

hearts of palm   Firm, elongated, off-white cylinders from the inside of a palm tree stem tip.

herbes de Provence   A seasoning mix of basil, fennel, marjoram, rosemary, sage, and thyme common in the south of France.

hoisin sauce   A sweet Asian condiment similar to ketchup made with soybeans, sesame, chile peppers, and sugar.

hors d'oeuvre   French for "outside of work" (the "work" being the main meal), an hors d'oeuvre can be any dish served as a starter before a meal.

horseradish   A sharp, spicy root that forms the flavor base in condiments such as cocktail sauce and sharp mustards. Prepared horseradish contains vinegar and oil, among other ingredients. Use pure horseradish much more sparingly than the prepared version, or try cutting it with sour cream.

hummus   A thick, Middle Eastern spread made of puréed chickpeas, lemon juice, olive oil, garlic, and often tahini.

infusion   A liquid in which flavorful ingredients such as herbs have been soaked or steeped to extract their flavor into the liquid.

isoflavone   A plant estrogen found in soybeans associated with reducing inflammation. Also called phytoestrogen.

Italian seasoning   A blend of dried herbs, including basil, oregano, rosemary, and thyme.

jicama   A juicy, crunchy, sweet, large, round Central American vegetable. If you can't find jicama, try substituting sliced water chestnuts.

julienne   A French word meaning "to slice into very thin pieces."

kalamata olive   Traditionally from Greece, a medium-small, long black olive with a rich, smoky flavor.

Key lime   A very small lime grown primarily in Florida known for its tart taste.

knead   To work dough to make it pliable so it holds gas bubbles as it bakes. Kneading is fundamental in the process of making yeast breads. Gluten-free breads often don't require as much, if any, kneading.

kosher salt   A coarse-grained salt made without any additives or iodine.

lacinto kale   A dark, leafy green kale. Also called Tuscan or dinosaur kale.

lentil   A tiny lens-shape bean used in European, Middle Eastern, and Indian cuisines.

local   Food grown, raised, or produced close to where you live, usually within a 100-mile radius, but that can be expanded to a region of one or two neighboring states.

locavore   A person who embraces and tries to eat local foods, often grown within a 100-mile radius of his or her home.

lysine   One of the 20 essential amino acids that provide the building blocks for human protein. Eight of the 20 are required for adults—isoleucine, leucine, lysine, methionine, phenylalanine, threonine, tryptophan, and valine. Grains usually don't contain much lysine, but amaranth and buckwheat do.

malabsorption   *See* nutritional malabsorption.

marinate   To soak meat, seafood, or another food in a seasoned sauce (a marinade) that's high in acid content. The acids break down the muscle of the meat, making it tender and adding flavor.

marjoram   A sweet herb, cousin of and similar to oregano popular in Greek, Spanish, and Italian dishes.

meld   To allow flavors to blend and spread over time. Melding is often why recipes call for overnight refrigeration and is also why some dishes taste better as leftovers.

meringue   A baked mixture of sugar and beaten egg whites, often used as a dessert topping.

mesclun   Mixed salad greens, usually containing lettuce and other assorted greens such as arugula, cress, and endive.

mesquite flour   A gluten-free flour made from the dried beans of the mesquite tree. It acts as a flour or as a spice, with its sweet and earthy, almost nutty flavor.

microgreens   Tiny, edible vegetables and herbs harvested when they're only 1 to $1^1/_2$ inches long with tiny green leaves. Long prized by chefs, they pack a wallop of a flavor for their size.

millet   A tiny, round, yellow-colored nutty-flavored grain often used as a replacement for couscous.

mince   To cut into very small pieces, smaller than diced, about $^1/_8$ inch or smaller.

mis en place   French term that means "everything in its place."

miso   A fermented, flavorful soybean paste, key in many Japanese dishes.

modified food starch   A starch that's altered in some way—sometimes even using chemicals. Often produced from a number of different substances, including wheat, it's frequently used as a thickener. According to FALCPA, the food's label must state if it's made from wheat. Starch and dextrin can also be made from wheat.

mouthfeel   The overall sensation in the mouth resulting from a combination of a food's temperature, taste, smell, and texture.

natural flavoring   A flavoring added to food; can be the essence of any product derived from food products. Don't assume *natural flavoring* means "gluten free"; many contain gluten.

nutmeg   A sweet, fragrant, musky spice used primarily in baking.

nutritional malabsorption   When your body—specifically your digestive tract—reacts to food by not absorbing its nutrients.

olive   The fruit of the olive tree commonly grown on all sides of the Mediterranean. Black olives are also called ripe olives. Green olives are immature, although they're also widely eaten. *See also* kalamata olives.

olive oil   A fragrant liquid produced by crushing or pressing olives. Extra-virgin olive oil—the most flavorful and highest quality—is produced from the first pressing of a batch of olives; oil is also produced from later pressings.

oregano   A fragrant, slightly astringent herb used in Greek, Spanish, and Italian dishes.

organic   A practice of farming that uses fewer pesticides, fertilizers, and other chemicals than standard farming.

orzo   A rice-shape pasta used in Greek cooking.

oxidation   The browning of fruit flesh that happens over time and with exposure to air. Minimize oxidation by rubbing the cut surfaces with lemon juice.

paella   A Spanish dish of rice, shellfish, onion, meats, rich broth, and herbs.

Paleo   A grain-free diet that incorporates fresh, whole foods.

pan-fry   To cook large pieces of food, with a little fat, over medium to medium-high heat, occasionally stirring or flipping.

panko   A large, coarse style of breadcrumbs. They're often used in Japanese cuisine, but more and more chefs and home cooks are using them in recipes that call for regular breadcrumbs. Look for gluten-free versions.

paprika   A rich, red, warm, earthy spice that lends a rich red color to many dishes.

parboil   To partially cook in boiling water or broth.

parsley   A fresh-tasting green leafy herb, often used as a garnish.

pâté   A savory loaf that contains meats, poultry, or seafood; spices; and often a lot of fat. It's served cold and spread or sliced on crusty bread or crackers.

pecan flour   A gluten-free flour, also called pecan meal, made from ground pecans. Pecan flour is nice in piecrusts and breads and can be used as a coating for meats.

pesto   A thick spread or sauce made with fresh basil leaves, garlic, olive oil, pine nuts, and Parmesan cheese.

pilaf   A rice dish in which the rice is browned in butter or oil and then cooked in a flavorful liquid such as a broth, often with the addition of meats or vegetables. The rice absorbs the broth, resulting in a savory dish.

pinch   An unscientific measurement for the amount of an ingredient—typically, a dry, granular substance such as an herb or seasoning—you can hold between your finger and thumb.

pine nut   A nut that's rich (high in fat), flavorful, and a bit pine-y. Pine nuts are a traditional ingredient in pesto and add a hearty crunch to many other recipes.

pita bread   A flat, hollow wheat bread often used for sandwiches or sliced pizza style. They're terrific soft with dips or baked or broiled as a vehicle for other ingredients. Look for gluten-free versions.

pizza stone   A flat stone that when preheated with the oven, cooks crusts to a crispy, pizza-parlor texture.

poach   To cook a food in simmering liquid such as water, wine, or broth.

polenta   A mush made from cornmeal that can be eaten hot with butter or cooked until firm and cut into squares.

porcini mushroom   A rich and flavorful mushroom used in rice and Italian-style dishes.

portobello mushroom   A mature and larger form of the smaller crimini mushroom. Brown, chewy, and flavorful, portobellos are often served as whole caps, grilled, or as thin sautéed slices. *See also* crimini mushrooms.

potato flour   A gluten-free flour, sometimes called potato starch flour, made from the entire cooked potato. It acts as a binder when used in baked goods. Use only in small amounts to avoid a final recipe that's gummy and heavy.

potato starch   A gluten-free thickening agent made from the starch of the potato. It has a fine, powdery texture and helps make gluten-free baked goods moister.

preheat   To turn on an oven, broiler, or other cooking appliance in advance of cooking so the temperature will be at the desired level when the assembled dish is ready for cooking.

prosciutto   A dry, salt-cured ham that originated in Italy.

protein   The collection of 20 amino acids the body requires for survival. A complete protein includes all 20 amino acids; an incomplete protein is missing one or more of the amino acids. Complementary proteins refer to foods that are incomplete proteins separately but provide an excellent protein when combined.

purée   To reduce a food to a thick, creamy texture, typically using a blender or food processor.

quinoa   A nutty-flavored gluten-free seed that's extremely high in protein and calcium.

reduce   To boil or simmer a broth or sauce to remove some of the water content, resulting in more concentrated flavor and color.

render   To cook a meat to the point where its fat melts and can be removed.

reserve   To hold a specified ingredient for another use later in the recipe.

rice vinegar   Vinegar produced from fermented rice or rice wine, popular in Asian-style dishes. (It's not the same thing as rice wine vinegar.)

risotto   A popular Italian rice dish made by browning arborio rice in butter or oil and then slowly adding liquid to cook the rice, resulting in a creamy texture.

roast   To cook something uncovered in an oven, usually without additional liquid.

rosemary   A pungent, sweet herb used with chicken, pork, fish, and especially lamb. A little goes a long way.

roux   A mixture of butter or another fat and flour used to thicken sauces and soups.

saffron   An expensive spice made from the stamens of crocus flowers. Saffron lends a dramatic yellow color and distinctive flavor to a dish. Use only tiny amounts.

sage   An herb with a musty yet fruity, lemon-rind scent and "sunny" flavor.

sauté   To pan-cook over lower heat than what's used for frying.

savory   A popular herb with a fresh, woody taste. Can also describe the flavor of food.

scald   To heat milk just until it's about to boil and then remove it from heat. Scalding milk helps prevent it from souring.

scant   An ingredient measurement directive not to add any extra, perhaps even leaving the measurement a tad short.

sea salt   Salt harvested from the sea.

sear   To quickly brown the exterior of a food, especially meat, over high heat.

sesame oil   An oil made from pressing sesame seeds. It's tasteless if clear and aromatic and flavorful if brown.

shallot   A member of the onion family that grows in a bulb somewhat like garlic but has a milder onion flavor. When a recipe calls for shallot, use the entire bulb.

shellfish   A broad range of seafood, including clams, mussels, oysters, crabs, shrimp, and lobster.

shiitake mushroom   A large, dark brown mushroom with a hearty, meaty flavor. It can be used fresh or dried, grilled, as a component in other recipes, and as a flavoring source for broth.

short-grain rice   A starchy rice popular in Asian-style dishes because it readily clumps, making it perfect for eating with chopsticks.

simmer   To boil a liquid gently so it barely bubbles.

skillet (also **frying pan**)   A generally heavy, flat-bottomed, metal pan with a handle designed to cook food over heat on a stovetop or campfire.

skim   To remove fat or other material from the top of liquid.

sorghum   A gluten-free cereal grain that's high in antioxidants.

soy flour   A gluten-free flour made from milling roasted soybeans that's rich in isoflavones. It's often used in baked goods and to help thicken gravies.

steam   To suspend a food over boiling water and allow the heat of the steam (water vapor) to cook the food. This quick-cooking method preserves a food's flavor and texture.

steep   To let sit in hot water, as in steeping tea in hot water for 10 minutes.

stew   To slowly cook pieces of food submerged in a liquid. Also, a dish prepared by this method.

sticky rice   *See* short-grain rice.

stir-fry   To cook small pieces of food in a wok or skillet over high heat, moving and turning the food quickly to cook all sides.

stock   A flavorful broth made by cooking meats and/or vegetables with seasonings until the liquid absorbs these flavors. The liquid is strained, and the solids are discarded. Stock can be eaten alone or used as a base for soups, stews, etc.

strata   A savory bread pudding made with eggs and cheese.

table salt   Finely ground salt or sodium chloride. It's often called iodized salt, but it doesn't necessarily contain iodine.

tahini   A paste made from sesame seeds used to flavor many Middle Eastern recipes.

tamari   A wheat-free soy sauce.

tamarind   A sweet, pungent, flavorful fruit used in Indian-style sauces and curries.

tapas   A Spanish term meaning "small plate" that describes individual-size appetizers and snacks served cold or warm.

tapenade   A thick, chunky spread made from savory ingredients such as olives, lemon juice, and anchovies.

tapioca starch   A gluten-free thickening agent, also called tapioca flour or cassava flour, that's great in foods with a high acid content, such as fruit pie fillings.

tarragon   A sweet, rich-smelling herb perfect with seafood, vegetables (especially asparagus), chicken, and pork.

teff   A tiny, darkish-red grain rich in calcium—1 cup grain contains 123 milligrams—and vitamin C.

tempeh   An Indonesian food made by culturing and fermenting soybeans into a cake, sometimes mixed with grains or vegetables. It's high in protein and fiber.

teriyaki   A Japanese-style sauce composed of soy sauce, rice wine, ginger, and sugar that works well with seafood as well as most meats.

thickening agent   A starch that changes the viscosity of liquids. A gluten-free thickening agent—such as arrowroot, cornstarch, or tapioca starch—helps bind together liquids or make baked goods taste lighter.

thyme   A minty, zesty herb.

tiramisu   An Italian dessert made from ladyfingers or a spongy cake soaked in coffee, layered with a mixture of mascarpone cheese and eggs, and topped with chocolate shavings.

tofu   A cheeselike substance made from soybeans and soy milk.

turmeric   A spicy, pungent yellow root used in many dishes, especially Indian cuisine, for color and flavor. Turmeric is the source of the yellow color in many prepared mustards.

tzatziki   A Greek dip traditionally made with Greek yogurt, cucumbers, garlic, and mint.

umami   The fifth taste, after sweet, salty, sour, and bitter.

vanillin   Artificial vanilla flavoring, not derived from real vanilla beans.

veal   Meat from a calf, generally characterized by its mild flavor and tenderness.

vegan   A person who consumes no animal products nor uses or wears any animal or insect by-products. Also refers to food made from no animal or insect products or by-products.

vegetable steamer   An insert with tiny holes in the bottom designed to fit on or in another pot to hold food to be steamed above boiling water. *See also* steam.

venison   Deer meat.

vinegar   An acidic liquid widely used as a dressing and seasoning, often made from fermented grapes, apples, or rice. *See also* balsamic vinegar; cider vinegar; rice vinegar; white vinegar; wine vinegar.

wasabi   Japanese horseradish, a fiery, pungent condiment used with many Japanese-style dishes. It's most often sold as a powder to which you add water to create a paste.

water chestnut   A white, crunchy, and juicy tuber popular in many Asian dishes. It holds its texture whether cool or hot.

whisk   To rapidly mix, introducing air to the mixture.

white mushroom   A button mushroom. When fresh, white mushrooms have an earthy smell and an appealing soft crunch.

white vinegar   The most common type of vinegar, produced from grain.

whole food   A food in its natural, unprocessed state. Fresh or frozen broccoli is a whole food, but broccoli with lemon pepper sauce or cheese sauce is not.

whole grain   A grain derived from the seeds of grasses, including rice, oats, rye, wheat, wild rice, quinoa, barley, buckwheat, bulgur, corn, millet, amaranth, and sorghum. Many whole grains contain gluten.

whole-bean flour   A robust gluten-free flour made from romano beans. It can be used in bread baking.

whole-wheat flour   Wheat flour that contains the entire grain.

wild rice   Not a rice at all, this grass has a rich, nutty flavor and serves as a nutritious side dish.

wine vinegar   Vinegar produced from red or white wine.

xanthan gum   A gluten-free thickening agent made from fermented corn sugar, or glucose. Xanthan gum helps give baked goods volume.

yeast   Tiny fungi that, when mixed with water, sugar, flour, and heat, release carbon dioxide bubbles, which, in turn, cause the bread to rise.

zest   Small slivers of peel, usually from a citrus fruit such as a lemon, lime, or orange.

Resources

We've scoured libraries, bookstores, and the internet to bring you even more resources to further your gluten-free lifestyle. So if you're interested in gluten-free baking, we have some recommendations. Feeling a little Paleo? We've got you covered there, too.

Books

As we moved toward gluten-free living, friends and doctors made recommendations for references that could help us. In our years of gluten-free living, we've studied a number of books to learn what we could about gluten and living well without gluten. Here are some books you might want to check out.

Agatston, Arthur. *The South Beach Diet Gluten Solution: The Delicious, Doctor-Designed, Gluten-Aware Plan for Losing Weight and Feeling Great—Fast!* New York: Rodale, 2013.

Ahern, Shauna James. *Gluten-Free Girl: How I Found the Food That Loves Me Back and How You Can, Too.* New Jersey: Wiley, 2007.

Amsterdam, Elana. *The Gluten-Free Almond Flour Cookbook.* New York: Celestial Arts, 2009.

———. *Gluten-Free Cupcakes.* New York: Celestial Arts, 2011.

———. *Paleo Cooking from Elana's Pantry.* Berkeley: Ten Speed Press, 2013.

Anca, Alexandra MHSc, RD, with Theresa Santandrea-Cull. *Complete Gluten-Free Diet and Nutrition Guide.* Toronto: Robert Rose, 2010.

Anderson, Jean. *The Nutrition Bible: A Comprehensive, No-Nonsense Guide to Foods, Nutrients, Additives, Preservatives, Pollutants, and Everything Else We Eat and Drink.* New York: William Morrow Cookbooks, 1997.

Beasley, Sandra. *Don't Kill the Birthday Girl: Tales from an Allergic Life.* New York: Broadway Paperbacks, 2011.

Blum, Susan S., with Michele Bender. *The Immune System Recovery Plan: A Doctor's 4-Step Program to Treat Autoimmune Disease.* New York: Scribner, 2013.

Compart, Pamela J. *The Kid-Friendly ADHD and Autism Cookbook: The Ultimate Guide to the Gluten-Free, Milk-Free Diet.* Beverly, MA: Fair Winds Press, 2012.

Epstein, Becky Sue. *Substituting Ingredients: The A to Z Kitchen Reference.* Guilford, CT: Globe Pequot, 1996.

Green, Peter H. R., MD, and Rory Jones. *Celiac Disease: A Hidden Epidemic, Revised Edition.* New York: William Morrow, 2010.

Greene, Bert. *The Grains Cookbook.* New York: Workman, 1989.

Halstead, Pauli. *Primal Cuisine: Cooking for the Paleo Diet.* Rochester, VT: Healing Arts Press, 2012.

Hasselbeck, Elisabeth. *The G-Free Diet: A Gluten-Free Survival Guide.* New York: Center Street, 2011.

Le Breton, Marilyn. *The AiA Gluten and Dairy Free Cook Book.* London: Jessica Kingsley, 2008.

Lieberman, Shari. *The Gluten Connection: How Gluten Sensitivity May Be Sabotaging Your Health—and What You Can Do to Take Control Now.* New York: Rodale, 2007.

Lowell, Jax Peters. *Against the Grain: The Slightly Eccentric Guide to Living Well Without Gluten or Wheat.* New York: Henry Holt & Company, 1996.

McGee, Harold. *On Food and Cooking: The Science and Lore of the Kitchen.* New York: Scribner, 1984.

McKenna, Erin. *BabyCakes: Vegan, Gluten-Free, and (Mostly) Sugar-Free Recipes from New York's Most Talked-About Bakery.* New York: Clarkson Potter, 2009.

O'Brien, Susan. *Gluten-Free, Sugar-Free Cooking.* New York: De Capo Press, 2008.

Roberts, Annalise G. *The Gluten-Free Good Health Cookbook: The Delicious Way to Strengthen Your Immune System and Neutralize Inflammation.* Evanston, IL: Surrey, 2009.

Ryberg, Roben. *The Gluten-Free Kitchen.* New York: Clarkson Potter, 2000.

Thompson, Tricia, MS, RD. *The Gluten-Free Nutrition Guide.* New York: McGraw-Hill, 2008.

Vartanian, Arsy. *The Paleo Slow Cooker: Healthy, Gluten-Free Meals the Easy Way.* New York: Race Point Publishing, 2013.

Wangen, Stephen. *Healthier Without Wheat: A New Understanding of Wheat Allergies, Celiac Disease, and Non-Celiac Gluten Intolerance.* Seattle: Innate Health Publishing, 2009.

Washburn, Donna, and Heather Butt. *The Gluten-Free Baking Book.* Toronto: Robert Rose, 2011.

Wills, Judith. *The Food Bible.* New York: Simon & Schuster Editions, 1998.

Wolf, Robb. *The Paleo Solution: The Original Human Diet.* Las Vegas: Victory Belt, 2010.

Magazines

These magazines offer recipes, topical info, and ideas for gluten-free eating. You may even find yourself subscribing to keep up on all things gluten free!

Delight Gluten Free Magazine
DelightGlutenFree.com

Easy Eats
easyeats.com

Gluten-Free Living
GlutenFreeLiving.com

Living Without and *Living Without's Gluten-Free Recipes and How To's*
LivingWithout.com

Simply Gluten Free Magazine
SimplyGlutenFreeMag.com

Blogs

Blogs are a fantastic way to learn about new recipes and be reminded that you're not alone. For more gluten-free blogs, check out CeliacCentral.org; click the Community tab and then Gluten-Free Bloggers.

Gluten Dude: The Naked Truth About Living Gluten Free
glutendude.com

The Healthy Apple: Your Guide to Clean Eating
thehealthyapple.com

Grub
thisisgrub.com
This site contains useful resources for those changing their eating habits.

Gluten Freely Frugal
glutenfreelyfrugal.com

Communities

Meeting others—even virtually—can help you as you transition to a gluten-free diet. Some manufacturers also provide forums for gluten-free folks, including a stable of bloggers.

BrainTalk Communities

braintalkcommunities.org/forum.php
Check out the Gluten Sensitivity/Celiac Disease community.

Udi's

udisglutenfree.com
This gluten-free bread maker's entire site is worth a look, but do check out the Community area and the coupons for bread products.

Rudi's

rudisbakery.com
Features bloggers and their gluten-free eating and lives.

Support Organizations

Sometimes a little helping hand can be useful. These organizations share a wealth of gluten-free information for you and can connect you with a wider community of gluten-free living.

American Celiac Disease Alliance

americanceliac.org
Also helps support 1in133.org, which advocates for the passage of clear labeling.

Canadian Celiac Association

celiac.ca

Celiac Disease Foundation

celiac.org

Celiac Sprue Association

csaceliacs.info

Gluten Free Calendar

glutenfreecalendar.com
Lists gluten-free events across the United States.

GlutenFreeFind.com

glutenfreefind.com
Provides American and Canadian resources.

Gluten Intolerance Group
gluten.net/local-branches

National Foundation for Celiac Awareness
CeliacCentral.org

National Institutes of Health Celiac Disease Awareness Campaign
celiac.nih.gov

Podcasts

Want to subscribe and listen to gluten-free living podcasts? A few are available on iTunes.

Gluten Free School Podcast with Jennifer Fugo

The Gluten Free Magazine Podcast (*The Gluten Free Magazine* is also available through iTunes.)

Hold the Gluten

Smartphone Apps

Gluten free doesn't mean mobile free. Get out and eat or shop with these mobile apps available for iPhones, Android phones, and various other smartphones via iTunes, Google Play, or Amazon. Apps come and go, so to keep updated on what apps are still available, log on to AppShopper (appshopper.com) and search for "gluten free." The Academy of Nutrition and Dietetics maintains a list of iPhone apps for gluten-free eating at bit.ly/145ehLC.

AllergyEats
allergyeats.com

Dine Gluten Free
glutenfreetravelsite.com

Find Me Gluten Free
www.findmeglutenfree.com

Gluten Free Ingredients
nations-software.info

Gluten Free Restaurant Cards
glutenfreepassport.com

Gluten Free Scanner
celiaccess.com

Gluten Free News
nations-software.info

Gluten-Free Groceries
triumphdining.com

Is That Gluten Free? For Groceries and
Is That Gluten Free? Eating Out
midlifecrisisapps.com

Product and Shopping Websites

Sometimes your local store is out of that gluten-free barbecue sauce or pasta you fell in love with. Or maybe you're planning a trip to Paris—how do you tell your waiter? Jump on the internet and find gluten-free products for everyday living at one of these gluten-friendly sites.

Abe's Market
abesmarket.com

Gluten Free/Allergy Free Travel Cards and Books
glutenfreepassport.com
Helps you travel the world without getting glutened.

The Gluten-Free Mall
celiac.com/glutenfreemall

GlutenSolutions.com
glutensolutions.com

LocalHarvest
localharvest.com
Find local farmers where you can purchase produce and meat.

Nielsen-Massey
nielsenmassey.com
A great place to order gluten-free vanillas and flavorings like peppermint or almond.

Penzeys Spices
penzeys.com
Shop here for gluten-free spices.

Red Apple Lipstick
redapplelipstick.com
Buy fashionable colors of gluten-free lipstick and other makeup here.

Spice House

thespicehouse.com

Another great place to shop for gluten-free spices.

Triumph Dining

triumphdining.com

Books and cards to help you navigate restaurants and grocery stores.

Product Delivery Websites

Check out these sites, where you can sign up to receive regular shipments of gluten-free foods.

GFree Connect

gfreeconnect.com

Enables you to select your preferences, including other allergens besides gluten. (However, please read the ingredients list for your own safety!) Also provides coupons for many of the products you order.

Sprig

sprigbox.com

Enables you to set up automatic, regular deliveries of a selection of full-size gluten-free foods. Does not have a system for separating foods that include other allergens.

Taste Guru

tasteguru.com

Provides automatic, monthly shipments of a variety of gluten-free foods.

Classes and Other Instructional Sites

Improve your cooking skills or learn some new recipes by checking out these sites.

Glutenfreeda

glutenfreeda.com

Gluten Free School with Jennifer Fugo

glutenfreeschool.com

YouTube.com

Search for "gluten-free cooking."

Testing

If you're unsure is something in your home has gluten in it, you can test it. Many of the online product sites also sell gluten-free testing kits you can use at home.

ELISA Technologies
elisa-tek.com
Offers an EZ Gluten kit you can use to test for gluten as low as 10 parts per million.

Medical and Research Organizations

Even if you've been diagnosed already, these sites are great for reading up on the latest research and gluten-free medical news.

Celiac Disease Center at Columbia University Medical Center
celiacdiseasecenter.org

Center for Celiac Research and Treatment
celiaccenter.org

The University of Chicago Celiac Disease Center
cureceliacdisease.org

William K. Warren Medical Research Center for Celiac Disease, University of California, San Diego
celiaccenter.ucsd.edu

Gluten-Free Shopping List

Throughout this book, we've given you lots of information on what to stock in your gluten-free kitchen. In this appendix, we cull all that info into a handy, grab-and-go list you can take with you to the store or make copies of and store on your pantry door so you can tick off the items you want to remember to pick up at the store.

For your pantry:

Breads, grains, and pastas:

- ❏ Brown rice
- ❏ Buckwheat groats
- ❏ Corn flake cereal
- ❏ Corn tortillas
- ❏ Gluten-free bagels
- ❏ Gluten-free bread
- ❏ Gluten-free crackers, regular or low-sodium
- ❏ Gluten-free English muffins
- ❏ Gluten-free graham crackers
- ❏ Gluten-free oats, old-fashioned or quick-cooking
- ❏ Gluten-free pasta in different shapes and sizes and made with different grains, such as quinoa, rice or a blend
- ❏ Gluten-free pretzels
- ❏ Grits
- ❏ Long-grain rice
- ❏ Polenta
- ❏ Quinoa
- ❏ Quinoa flake cereal
- ❏ Rice cakes
- ❏ Rice cereal, hot and cold
- ❏ Teff tortillas
- ❏ _____
- ❏ _____
- ❏ _____
- ❏ _____
- ❏ _____

Pure spices and seasonings:

- ❏ Black pepper
- ❏ Cayenne
- ❏ Cinnamon
- ❏ Crushed red pepper flakes
- ❏ Garlic chile sauce or hot sauce
- ❏ Garlic powder
- ❏ Gluten-free premixed seasonings
- ❏ Ground ginger
- ❏ Ketchup
- ❏ Minced onion
- ❏ Mustard
- ❏ Nutmeg
- ❏ Onion powder
- ❏ Paprika
- ❏ _____
- ❏ _____
- ❏ _____
- ❏ _____
- ❏ _____

Baking:

- ❏ All-purpose gluten-free flour
- ❏ Baking powder
- ❏ Baking soda
- ❏ Brown rice flour
- ❏ Brown sugar
- ❏ Chocolate syrup
- ❏ Gluten-free cornstarch
- ❏ Gluten-free icing
- ❏ Gluten-free pancake and waffle mixes
- ❏ Gluten-free pastry flour

❑ Gluten-free pizza mixes

❑ Gluten-free vanilla extract

❑ Granulated sugar

❑ Honey

❑ Peanut butter (read label)

❑ Semisweet chocolate chips

❑ Yeast, except brewer's yeast

❑ _____

❑ _____

❑ _____

❑ _____

❑ _____

Oils, sauces, and dressings:

❑ Canola oil

❑ Cider vinegar

❑ Gluten-free barbecue sauces

❑ Gluten-free gravy mixes

❑ Gluten-free hoisin sauce

❑ Gluten-free rice vinegar

❑ Gluten-free soy sauce

❑ Gluten-free tamari sauce

❑ Gluten-free teriyaki sauce

❑ Oil spray (baking spray may contain gluten)

❑ Olive oil

❑ White vinegar

❑ _____

❑ _____

❑ _____

❑ _____

❑ _____

Beverages:

- ❏ Coffee (check labels if flavored)
- ❏ Gluten-free beer
- ❏ Gluten-free juices
- ❏ Soda
- ❏ Tea (check label if flavored)
- ❏ Wine
- ❏ _____
- ❏ _____
- ❏ _____
- ❏ _____
- ❏ _____

Fresh fruits and vegetables:

- ❏ Apples
- ❏ Avocados
- ❏ Bananas
- ❏ Broccoli
- ❏ Green beans
- ❏ Lettuce
- ❏ Onions or green onions
- ❏ Oranges
- ❏ Peaches
- ❏ Peas
- ❏ Pears
- ❏ Pineapple
- ❏ Potatoes
- ❏ Sweet potatoes
- ❏ Pumpkin
- ❏ Tomatoes
- ❏ _____
- ❏ _____
- ❏ _____

❏ _____

❏ _____

Canned goods without sauces:

❏ Broth or bouillon for chicken stock

❏ Broth or bouillon for beef stock

❏ Broth or bouillon for vegetable stock

❏ Canned beans

❏ Canned tomatoes

❏ Canned fish (without sauces)

❏ Soups (read label)

❏ _____

❏ _____

❏ _____

❏ _____

❏ _____

Dried fruit:

❏ Dried apples

❏ Dried apricots

❏ Dried bananas

❏ Dried cherries

❏ Dried cranberries

❏ Dried peaches

❏ Dried pineapple

❏ Dried strawberries

❏ Raisins

❏ _____

❏ _____

❏ _____

❏ _____

❏ _____

Nuts:

- ❏ Almonds
- ❏ Brazil nuts
- ❏ Cashews
- ❏ Hazelnuts
- ❏ Macadamia nuts
- ❏ Peanuts
- ❏ Pecans
- ❏ Pine nuts
- ❏ Pistachios
- ❏ Walnuts
- ❏ _____
- ❏ _____
- ❏ _____
- ❏ _____
- ❏ _____

For your refrigerator:

- ❏ Butter
- ❏ Canned or jarred olives
- ❏ Cheese
- ❏ Cream cheese (with flavors, read label)
- ❏ Deli meats (read label)
- ❏ Gluten-free salad dressing
- ❏ Gluten-free hot dogs
- ❏ Gluten-free sausages
- ❏ Jams
- ❏ Jellies
- ❏ Large eggs
- ❏ Marmalades
- ❏ Mayonnaise
- ❏ Meat (unprocessed meats are safe)
- ❏ Milk

- ❑ Plain Greek yogurt
- ❑ Plain or vanilla yogurt (with flavors, read label)
- ❑ Seafood (with sauces, read label)
- ❑ Sour cream (with flavors, read label)
- ❑ _____
- ❑ _____
- ❑ _____
- ❑ _____
- ❑ _____

For your freezer:

- ❑ Gluten-free breakfast meats
- ❑ Gluten-free frozen cinnamon rolls
- ❑ Gluten-free frozen dinners (read label)
- ❑ Gluten-free frozen doughnuts
- ❑ Gluten-free frozen entrées (read label)
- ❑ Gluten-free frozen pizzas (read label)
- ❑ Gluten-free frozen sides (read label)
- ❑ Gluten-free frozen waffles
- ❑ Ice cream (check label)
- ❑ _____
- ❑ _____
- ❑ _____
- ❑ _____
- ❑ _____

Frozen fruits and vegetables (without sauces):

- ❑ Apples
- ❑ Bananas
- ❑ Berries
- ❑ Broccoli
- ❑ Brussels sprouts

- ❏ Carrots
- ❏ Green beans
- ❏ Peaches
- ❏ Peas
- ❏ Pears
- ❏ Pineapple
- ❏ Potatoes
- ❏ _____
- ❏ _____
- ❏ _____
- ❏ _____
- ❏ _____

Gluten-Free Food Log

One way to track your reactions to new foods you eat while transitioning to a gluten-free diet is to keep a log. Be sure to note when and what you ate or drank, including how much you ingested and if you had any symptoms. You also might want to indicate if you'd buy the item again.

Meal	Food/Drink Consumed	Brand	Amount	Symptoms/ Reactions	Buy Again?
Breakfast					
Lunch					

Meal	Food/Drink Consumed	Brand	Amount	Symptoms/ Reactions	Buy Again?
Dinner					
Snack					

Index

Q-R

S